The safe word is Pineapple!

MAYOR TO MANIC - MY JOURNEY THROUGH CRAZY

GERRY TAFT

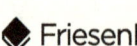 **FriesenPress**

One Printers Way
Altona, MB R0G 0B0
Canada

www.friesenpress.com

Copyright © 2024 by Gerry Taft
First Edition — 2024

All rights reserved.

No part of this publication may be reproduced in any form, or by any means, electronic or mechanical, including photocopying, recording, or any information browsing, storage, or retrieval system, without permission in writing from FriesenPress.

ISBN
978-1-03-831681-3 (Hardcover)
978-1-03-831680-6 (Paperback)
978-1-03-831682-0 (eBook)

1. BIOGRAPHY & AUTOBIOGRAPHY, PERSONAL MEMOIRS

Distributed to the trade by The Ingram Book Company

Introduction

WHY WRITE THE BOOK?

This book is about my mental/emotional meltdown in the fall of 2023. It is part memoir and part manifesto. A weird little book about a weird little guy from a weird little town.

Initially, during a very manic phase, I wanted to create a text that would be a "compassion bomb"—a disruptive explosion of love—and real talk that could empower "grey" (imperfect people) to lead with love and compassion, drop shame and guilt, call bullshit on broken systems, and work to improve themselves, their families, and their communities. But realistically, I'll settle for it being a kind of interesting read that breaks down a bit of stigma and generates a bit of thought or conversation.

There are friends, family, and others who would like to forget about my breakdown and pretend it never happened. There are work colleagues (and probably political advisors if I had any) who would recommend deleting any past social media posts from that time, advise against recounting the experience, and recommend presenting a polished, squeaky clean public persona.

When I thought I was going to die, when I thought I had to pick between "good" and "evil," I made a pledge to a higher power to be a better person and to share my experience and learnings. At the time, writing a book seemed like a matter of life or death. Afterwards, it became therapeutic to try to make sense of what happened and to sort through the emotions of being "cancelled."

Later the book seemed like a terrible idea. Some advice from the owner of my former real estate brokerage rang through my ears a few times: "Mental health isn't just taking medication for a little bit and then you're cured." It is true. I haven't struggled with mental health for years, or decades, like many others have. I am not a subject expert.

But I know that telling my story from my perspective helps me to feel more understood. One could argue that this is self-serving, a PR spin. One could argue that I am self absorbed. This is all true. But I believe that I might not be the only person out there who can feel misunderstood, who craves for honesty, transparency, and real talk.

When it all felt too much, I asked for help. I posted on social media, I sought medical attention, and I leaned on family, friends, and community. I used my safe word. And miracles happened. There were people there to listen. It wasn't always what I wanted, and at times it felt like it was barely enough, but, ultimately, it was enough. I am here to tell the story!

I wrote this book because I refused to suffer in silence—and I don't think you should either! Thank you deeply to those who care; those who are listening, reading, thinking, and discussing mental health, society, and community.

CHAPTER 1
False Alarm

On the morning of Saturday, September 23rd, sitting in the familiar hotel restaurant in Calgary, I felt dizzy. Waves of thick fog were rolling over me. I had tried the day before at the Vancouver airport, the night before in the hotel room, and now this morning. I stared at my laptop, the words blurry, the details and dates fuzzy. I had done the work hundreds of times over the last 5 years as a successful realtor—but no matter how hard I pushed myself, no matter how guilty I felt for not doing it, I could not focus.

I wasn't hungry, but I knew that I should eat. I was impatient and snappy, small decisions were so difficult to make, ordering the meal was difficult. I didn't care what food I got. Why couldn't the server just leave me alone? Why was he so awkward and asking me so many questions?

The night before, I had struggled to book the hotel, to navigate technology and roads. I had booked this dumpy place to save $20, and then I had tipped the front desk girl $100 because I couldn't get the room card to work.

Last night I'd been pacing the hotel room and writing a book in my head, trying to solve the problems of society, trying to understand why there is so much homelessness, so much mental illness, polarization, so many conspiracy theories—why things seemed to be getting worse, so quickly. I knew that I was spinning. I knew my social interactions were getting weirder.

So much of me wanted the unravelling to be quick. *Maybe I can just be crazy this weekend and back to work on Monday? Maybe this will be the fastest nervous breakdown ever?* I really wanted that to be true.

At first, pacing the room the night before had been fun. My thoughts were profound, it felt like I was close to some big epiphanies, to some solutions, I was writing a book or a keynote speech in my head. *Maybe the solution was that the Union of British Columbia Municipalities needed a secret fraternity to make changes at the local government level happen faster? Maybe if I put all these amazing ideas into a book, it could change the world?*

But it shifted from being fun to this feeling of spinning, struggling to keep a grasp on what was real. I tried sleeping. One-hour increments. I would wake, document the time and a thought onto a piece of paper, hoping for the morning, hoping to be normal again.

Now that it was morning, I couldn't handle the restaurant, the fog, the spinning, the dread, the guilt. I wanted to run back up to the hotel room and stay there, hide there, write a book in one weekend, solve all of the problems . . .

But I forced myself to concentrate, to really focus on what mattered. The answer that came back crystal clear: *"See your kids one last time before you DIE."*

I don't know where that answer came from, but it made so much sense in the moment. I was going to end up in a hospital in Calgary or dying in that hotel room or dying on the drive home. These potential realities were close, I could sense them.

I asked myself, *How do I get home to see my kids?* And a voice inside me said: *"You know what to do. You just need to do it."*

I typed into my laptop simple instructions:

Finish your coffee

Pay the bill

Leave the restaurant

Phone a crisis help line

Drive home

I needed to talk to a human so badly, but not that annoying server, he was in my way, he was slowing me on my mission. It seemed like he was stopping me.

The fog in my brain was so thick, and there was literal fog outside. Everything was fucking symbolic, and everything felt like death.

I struggled to find the exit from the restaurant. I googled a number for a crisis helpline, the Bluetooth kicked in, the automated message was asking for my Alberta Health Care Card number, I'm from BC, I don't have a fucking Alberta Health number. Why was everything so hard to navigate? But there was a workaround. I finally got connected to a live agent. She wasn't friendly, she had a checklist of questions, and she was very focused on whether I was going to harm myself or someone else.

My eyes filled with tears, and I burst with emotion. It was so hard to admit that I was losing my mind. I didn't know what was happening. Never before in my life had I ever had the need to phone a crisis helpline. Never before in my life had I felt like I was losing my mind. Never before in my life did I feel such a lack of control. Never before in my life did it feel like the world was so against me.

The operator asked me if I was suicidal. It broke me and it hurt me to admit that I was 1% suicidal. Not because I wanted to die, but because the pressure, the pressure in my head, the fog around me, the pressure of the situation, the unexplainable dread of what was coming next, the fear of getting locked up in a psych ward in Calgary, the shame of disappointing everyone, my family, my clients, my office, myself. The feelings were so terrible, so strong, and so foreign to me, it felt almost unbearable.

But what was happening?

Rationally, admitting that I was 1% suicidal opened up some real fear: If I was cracking from 0% to 1%, that could be a really slippery slope.

Part of me knew this wasn't right. *I am not suicidal. Why do I even feel 1%? I have a great life, and my whole life is in front of me. To kill myself would make no sense at all, it isn't what I want. Why does it seem like "the world" or something is trying to make me think like this?*

I had to stay focused on driving to Invermere. The crisis helpline operator said I shouldn't be driving. I didn't disagree with her, but I had a single mission and purpose: I had to see my kids again. I missed a turn onto Stoney Trail, I asked for driving directions, she wouldn't give them to me. I thought to myself, *Some help line this is!* I still had a sense of humour. I smiled at my own joke.

It seemed like cars were cutting in front of me, that everything was pushing against me, trying to prevent me from leaving the city. So many things were going wrong, but I decided to view them as being humorous instead of getting angry or scared. I chuckled. *I don't care, it doesn't matter, cut me off, it doesn't matter, I have a mission, I have a sole focus, I know what to do, I will find the workarounds.*

I drove past Calaway Park on the outskirts of Calgary. The pressure, brain fog, and literal fog were lifting just slightly. The crisis helpline operator was ending the call. She suggested that I see a counsellor, and that maybe I was having a work-related nervous breakdown. I think she thought I wasted her time. I didn't care. It was what I needed, just barely enough to help me get out of the city.

Escaping the city had seemed like an impossible task, but now that I was out, I felt some freedom, a glimmer of hope. I turned on the satellite radio and turned up the electronic music, but after two minutes of vibrations and synthetic beats I phoned my best friend Justin, who hates electronic music. He answered and started having a totally normal conversation. I tried to explain that I wasn't normal, but I also loved trying to have a normal conversation and having real human connection. After the conversation ended, I switched the radio to comedy.

Comedian Chelsea Handler had an amazingly raw, sad but funny story titled "Loss/Abandonment." It's about her brother dying during her childhood, the reaction from her parents, the guilt it caused her, and how it screwed her up with men and relationships (she made jokes about wanting to hook up with her therapist). Everything she said made so much sense to me, it was so touching, it was exactly what I needed to hear in the moment. It was so human. The themes of death and guilt were so relevant to me. It was incredible. It seemed like a little miracle. It kept me going.

The closer I got to Invermere, the better I felt, almost normal. The brain fog slowly lifted, I was going to make it, I was actually going to make it.

Around 12:30 p.m., I made it home. I walked into my house, where my wife and kids were chilling on a lazy Saturday. As soon as I entered our home, I burst into tears. I hugged my kids, and I looked them in the eyes. It all made sense. For the first time in my life, I understood my own children.

Kelvin has anxiety. I had never experienced anxiety before, so I couldn't relate, but now I had felt it. I knew what it feels like for him. I understood him so much better.

Veronica hates being told what to do and is constantly pushing boundaries. Although she is a good person, deep down a caring person, she can be very annoying. I realized I can be like that too, that's how I must make some people feel.

I saw myself, my flaws, and my strengths in my children. I had a flood of childhood memories. It felt like I could access all of my memories. I finally understood myself, I finally understood my children, I finally understood the world and my place in it.

I knew that my wife and I didn't have the most affectionate relationship and that neither of us wanted to talk about relationship issues, but now there was urgency. I had no fear and no filter. Things I never thought I would say, or might take years to get the courage to discuss, I blurted out. I barfed out my faults and tried to pinpoint our relationship problems, all at once, to my stunned and tired wife. I was ready to blow up the marriage if that was necessary. Maybe that was what this was all about? She responded with calmness. She knew I wasn't acting normally. She listened.

I felt some peace, I felt some happiness. I felt comfortable and so grateful to have made it home. Maybe I could take a few days to heal at home and everything would go back to normal...

MORNING, SUNDAY, SEPTEMBER 24TH, INVERMERE

My heart was pounding, and my vision was blurry. I had felt this for the first time the day before in Calgary, but now it hit me even stronger and rolled in even faster, like a wave of evil energy, brain fog, an unshakable feeling of dread. I blurted out: "I need to go" as I quickly left our home, the home I had fought so hard to make it back to the day before.

I entered the Invermere hospital, the same hospital I was born in, in the same town that I'd been mayor of for ten years, choking back tears, filled with shame and embarrassment, in front of a bunch of people in the ER waiting room (who I probably knew but couldn't bear to look at). I told the admissions clerk, still choking back those shame-filled tears, "I am having some kind of mental health crisis . . . I need help."

She told me to find the button near the secure doors to the ER and to push the button and talk into the camera, and a nurse would buzz open the door.

I couldn't find the button, it wasn't right beside the door, I struggled to find the stupid button. I couldn't concentrate. Why was everything so complicated?

The young nurse was calm, kind, and pretty. She held my hand and touched my arm. She did her best to calm me down. Normally, I would have been self-conscious, but I accepted the human touch and compassion completely.

I started to tell the story: "I think I'm having some kind of mental breakdown. I don't know why. Maybe work, but not just work. I just attended the Union of British Columbia Municipalities Convention in Vancouver and have been away from home for a week, I didn't see my kids for a week, I had to make it home to see them . . ."

She asked how old my kids were, I struggled to remember. "My son, ah, he's . . . he's, ah, seven, no eight." Guilt came rushing in. What kind of piece-of-shit father doesn't know how old his son is?

I continued to ramble on. "I don't know what happened, but I experienced some weird shit. There is so much wrong with society right now: the wealth gap, homelessness is getting worse. On Thursday night, a small group of us went to this night club, it was for really rich people and it seemed kind of evil, I don't know why we were there—and then things just got weirder and weirder . . . we ended up at this Burger King full of homeless people . . ."

She stopped me. She gently told me she had to fill out this intake form and that she had other duties and other patients. She asked if I had any personal or family history of mental illness.

"No, not at all," I answered, thinking of myself and very immediate family (I forgot that some cousins on both sides have had struggles).

She asked if I was on any drugs.

"I have been vaping some marijuana recently, but no, I don't think I am on any other drugs, although this guy at the creepy club, I think he got drugged..."

All I wanted to do was tell the story, explain what I had experienced, and try to make sense of it. All I wanted was for someone to listen.

But no one had time to listen.

The nurse guided me toward a secure padded room near the end of the ER. Years earlier, when I had served on the East Kootenay Regional Hospital board and fought to get the provincial funding for the emergency room redevelopment, I remembered the plans included two secure psychiatric rooms near the edge of the ER.

Hell no, I thought. *I don't know what is happening but I'm not going into a room like that.* I had the distinct feeling that if I ended up in there, I might not ever get out. The last thing in the world I wanted was to be locked up.

I politely resisted. "No, I don't feel comfortable going in there."

Some other nurses got involved and they found me a non-padded room. I was left alone for a bit to stew in my thoughts, they took some blood, I peed into a cup (I remember being really happy to pee into the cup because I actually had to pee).

My wife had told my mom that I was acting weird and had gone to the hospital. My mom showed up. Initially I said I didn't want to see her, then I changed my mind. I wanted her to get my laptop from home. If no one had time to listen to me, at least I could write about what I was thinking and experiencing. Trying to document things had helped me a bit Friday night when I was spinning out of control in the hotel room in Calgary.

The Safe Word is PINEAPPLE!

But even my own mom wasn't listening. She was lingering around, asking me dumb questions and not getting my laptop (objectively, I think she was worried and trying to figure out what was going on). She was wasting time, she was making excuses, and she was making things complicated. I couldn't explain the urgency, but time really mattered, and she was wasting time.

"It doesn't fucking matter. Can you just go get the laptop please? No one is listening to me, I need that laptop," I snapped.

Sitting in the Invermere hospital, it slowly occurred to me: I was dying. Something was letting me know that my end was near. It explained the clarity, the understanding, the dread. It all made sense . . .

And what a fucking rip off!

To finally understand my kids and life, to finally be in a financial position to not have to work so hard, to finally have a little pontoon boat that I had struggled to pick up in August and was determined to use with friends and family or, if no one else wanted to go, to use by myself, to suddenly die at 41—it wasn't fair.

I told a nurse and my mom that I thought I might be dying. They asked me if I wanted to die.

"Absolutely not. I don't know why I am dying, I don't want to die." (Thankfully, I was 0% suicidal at that moment).

I wanted to be rushed to Cranbrook for a CT scan to see if I had an aggressive brain tumour, but it was a Sunday afternoon in Invermere and no one else thought I was dying and no one wanted to listen to me. Being white, male, middle class (maybe even upper middle class now), a community leader and on town council since I was 20 years old, and now not being believed and not being heard, not being listened to—I wasn't used to that. It was a frustrating feeling.

I knew there was no point in getting angry. If there was some crazy brain tumour, they probably couldn't do anything for me in Cranbrook anyway.

I thought about my kids. They are smart, and their mom is a good person and a good mother. If I died, it would be rough for them, but financially they would be secure enough. It would be better if I could be there for them growing up, but, ultimately, I knew they were going to turn out well. They were going to grow up to be good people.

I didn't want to die bitter. If death was actually happening, I had to accept it and I had to "get busy dying." While I could, I had to share what I had experienced in Vancouver, I had to share what I was feeling about society. There was something significant about that creepy night club in Vancouver—I didn't have all of the answers, I didn't understand it—but if I left some clues for others—little breadcrumbs of information—other people could figure it out and make sense of it all, and at least I wouldn't be dying for no reason. This gave me some peace, and it gave me focus on organizing a good death and telling my story while I could.

I sent emails and text messages to a few people, I made amends to a few people, I told a few people that I thought I was dying. It was so hard to do, but I reached out to the owner of my real estate office to say that I couldn't function in real estate and others would need to pick up the pieces.

I asked my sister to bring me Chinese buffet take out for my last meal. I asked my wife to bring the kids to the hospital so that I could say goodbye to them.

While I was trying to organize the best death possible, annoying people were sending annoying messages. A high-maintenance lady looking for a house sent a snarky note about how unprofessional it was that she had not heard from me in two days, an agent from Golden who couldn't figure out a lockbox on an already conditionally-sold home had phoned and texted numerous times. I couldn't deal with them, I couldn't waste what little time I had left on earth with their problems.

The Safe Word is PINEAPPLE!

I wanted to lash out at these people—tell them I was dying and they were wrecking my death—but I knew it wasn't their fault. The irony wasn't lost on me; I could see some humour in it. One of the last messages I might see could be from one of these annoying people. I couldn't get away from them, from work, from annoying people, even on my literal death bed.

My sister and her husband arrived with the Chinese food, and I asked my sister to film me talking. I started to ramble on. It felt good to tell my story and to be listened to. I was hungry but I only took one bite of ginger beef. I continued to talk with another piece of ginger beef dangling from my plastic fork. I wanted to eat but it would take away time from talking, and I also didn't want my death to come from choking on ginger beef. I love ginger beef. That would just be too unfair.

My wife arrived with the kids, and we paused on filming. It was hard not to cry, it was hard to say good bye to them. They didn't know I was dying, they just knew Daddy was acting a bit weird and in a hospital for some reason. I knew they didn't want to come into the hospital and they didn't want to see me in a hospital bed. I was so proud of them for coming.

I often fall asleep beside my beautiful little 5-year-old daughter, Veronica. She gave me her little penguin stuffy to cuddle (instead of her). It was so fucking beautiful.

My kids left the hospital room, my sister started to film again, I was about to talk about the creepy club in Vancouver and what I experienced on that Thursday night, but things had escalated. Now that I had said goodbye to my kids, things were speeding up . . .

I could feel death in my stomach.

Part of me was ready. I had done what I could, I could cuddle this penguin and I could just let go, but I didn't want to, it didn't feel right. I was going to keep talking until I couldn't . . .

My heart was pounding, I felt so much energy inside me. Death was crawling up into my throat, my heart was pounding, it was really happening . . .

BRRRRR-innngggg . . . *BRRRR-inggggg* . . . *BRRR-ingggg* . . .

THE FIRE ALARM WENT OFF.

My body shook in reaction to the sound. It took a second to process.

I wasn't dead.

My sister was still filming me.

"That is fucking weird, that is so weird."

I grabbed my wallet and started walking out of the room. "This is straight out of a fucking horror movie. I have an urge to leave."

A nurse called from down the hall: "It's from the care home next door. It's a false alarm."

False alarm indeed.

I told my sister and her husband to keep filming and to follow me out of the hospital. "There is no way I am staying here, it isn't safe, and there is no way they should stop me from leaving."

I had accepted a natural death. I didn't understand it and I wasn't happy about it, but I was as ready as I was going to be. But now it was clear: Someone or something was trying to kill me—or trick me into somehow choosing to die—and I didn't want anything to do with it.

Something wasn't right.

This was bigger than just me.

CHAPTER 2
Before

I was born on a Tuesday in the middle of June in 1982. My mom is proud to say she finished payroll (for the local NAPA Auto Parts store that her and my father owned) before driving herself to the Invermere hospital to give birth to me.

One of the earliest pieces of wisdom I remember from my dad: "Employees are lazy." I didn't even know what an employee was, but I knew I didn't want to be one of them. From an early age, I was dreaming up business ideas.

At the age of eight, I had big plans to open a store that sold Lego and had a Coke pop machine (combining my two loves at the time). I had to start small and raise some money, so I taped one yellow Kleenex box filled with Lego pieces to my desk in Mrs. Askey's Grade 3 classroom. Beside that I placed a smaller box with a slot for coins, and written details on the future amazing Lego store I'd soon be opening, with instructions, "Take a piece of Lego, leave a coin."

I decided it would be bad luck to check the progress of my Lego sales until the last day of school. I opened the boxes to find almost all of the Lego pieces gone and very little money in the money box. It was very disappointing, a true business setback. To make things worse, in trying to pack up my little Lego store, I missed the school bus.

My first elected office was Grade 5 class council. In Grades 6 and 7, I got really interested in federal politics, and I was proud to put a "Reform Party" bumper sticker onto my bike. When I was 14, I had the opportunity to travel to Ottawa and get a tour of the Parliament buildings with my local MP. When I was 16, I started attending British Columbia Youth Parliament (BCYP), an incredible organization where I met a lot of amazing people, started some romantic relationships, and developed lifelong friendships and connections.

After several different business schemes and ideas, my first real business was a hotdog cart that I started when I was 17 (and just beginning Grade 12). On the first day of grilling hotdogs and bratwurst in front of the Invermere Home Hardware store (when it used to be downtown), I was shaking with nervousness. I was afraid that someone would confront me and tell me that I didn't know what I was doing. But I faked it until I made it, and I sold out of product that first day.

After graduating high school, I enrolled in a 2-year tourism/hospitality management diploma program at what is now Thompson Rivers University in Kamloops. During those two years I learned a lot, but one of the most important lessons was during a tour of an Earls restaurant. The restaurant manager talked about the long hours she worked, and I noticed a fellow in the background sipping on a glass of wine. She introduced him. "This is Steve, the owner." Many of my classmates were going to work for big hotel chains. I felt a pull to small business. And I knew in that exact moment I didn't want to be the manager; I wanted to be the owner.

I also realized how much I missed my hometown of Invermere. During the time I lived in Kamloops, I would make my mom send me the local newspaper, *The Valley Echo*. I followed District of Invermere council meeting agendas and minutes online. And every time I went home to visit, I was excited to see what had changed in my town and I felt a bit sad to leave. Most of my high school friends were not coming back to Invermere, but I felt the pull home.

After graduating from college in the fall of 2002 and moving back full time to Invermere, I knew that I wanted to get involved in the municipal elections. Like the cheesy "No Fear" shirts of the 1990s, I really believed, "You are either part of the solution or part of the problem." I didn't want to be someone who complained on the sidelines; I wanted to be involved in making my hometown the best it could be. There were nine of us running for four council seats, and I was lucky to get in fourth. My campaign flyer had a picture of me holding a beer. Digital cameras weren't the norm. I had to find a physical photo, cut and tape it into my flyer and photocopy that, and it was the only photo I could find of myself. I figured, since I was only 20, I should just embrace it. My mom thought it would make me lose.

My girlfriend at the time, who I met through BCYP, introduced me to gelato during a trip to Vancouver. It was amazing, so smooth and fresh, so different than regular ice cream, and I knew that Invermere needed this and I would be the person to do this. This would be my business. I had two summers with a less successful traditional ice cream shop in a bad location in nearby Fairmont Hot Springs. After months of planning, physical renovations, a lot of painting, being rejected for business loans, and literally maxing out more than twenty credit cards and lines of credit and borrowing $30,000 from a retired couple, I opened Gerry's Gelati in downtown Invermere on May 3rd, 2004.

I noticed in the fall of 2004 and spring 2005 that real estate prices in Invermere were starting to rise. I feared not getting into the market. I made a deal with a local contractor to purchase an empty building lot in the Althamere section of Invermere: I had to pay him $40,000 by the end of the summer of 2005. It was stressful, but I was motivated, and it was a busy summer at the gelati shop. I scraped together the money. But then in the fall of 2005, shortly after buying the building lot, a little house behind Sobeys came up for sale. I could keep one bedroom for myself and rent out the rest of the rooms to Panorama Mountain Resort staff and cover the full mortgage costs—plus, it had a great backyard and a small garage that I could convert into a production kitchen for gelato. Although it seemed like a long shot, I was able to refinance the building lot and use that money for a downpayment on the house behind Sobeys. By the fall 2005, I was starting my new passion for leveraged real estate investing.

I used every dollar I earned, along with refinancing properties and some creative vendor financing deals, to buy more properties. The local real estate market was depressed from approximately 2010 to 2016, and during that time I was able to capitalize on some amazing deals, including buying two condos in foreclosure and a shut-down mini golf course/commercial building in Radium Hot Springs.

Near the beginning of 2008, the then -mayor of Invermere told the other council members that he wasn't going to run in the November municipal election. We all looked around the table at each other to see who would do it. At first, I didn't want to. It was a lot of work, and I was working at least 80 hours a week in my business, often staying up all night to make gelati. But I knew deep down that I could do it. It wasn't clear that anyone else on council wanted to run or had the skills. I didn't particularly crave the title, I wasn't sure I was ready for it, but I was fearful of who might try to run with no council experience. I felt obligated to use my experience and my skills and step up. I was elected as mayor in the fall of 2008 at the age of 26.

I was still a 26-year-old, single at the time, working long hours and going to the local bar on Friday and Saturday nights. The week after the election, someone came up to me at the bar and said, "What are you doing here?"

Some people talked to me more, some people were nicer to me, but there were also people watching everything I did or said more closely. I felt I was the same person as I'd always been, but I realized that the way a lot of people looked at me had changed.

The policy and the decision-making, the time spent on the Regional District of East Kootenay (RDEK) board, were enjoyable and engaging; however, I never felt completely comfortable or really enjoyed the ceremonial aspect of the position, such as parades, ribbon cuttings, or attending functions and meetings where the only purpose was to be there as a dignitary/figure head. I think that aspect of the position is better suited for someone older.

DEER CULL

One of the most controversial issues during my time as mayor was urban deer. After much study, discussion, and public process, the decision was made to do a limited and controlled cull of urban deer. It was a non-issue in the November 2011 municipal election, but immediately after I won a second term, a small but very vocal group formed and opposed the cull. It blew up on social media in late 2011 and early 2012.

There was a billboard on the highway about the deer cull cruelty, a lawsuit against the town attacked the public process (that was eventually dismissed), there were a few rallies, full-page newspaper ads that attacked me and council members. There was an attempt to organize a boycott of my business, some people online suggested that council members, not the deer, should be the ones killed. This nasty and polarizing debate went on for several years.

In 2013, after continuing to hear from the anti-cull people that they represented the silent majority of residents, we did an opinion poll (nonbinding referendum vote) on the topic, along with a referendum on borrowing money for a new community centre. Despite a huge effort from anti-cull folks to mobilize their vote, most people voted "yes" to deer culls as a tool to manage urban deer (729 to 259). After the vote, a number of deer traps were vandalized, first in Cranbrook. In February of 2014, the lead spokesperson for the anti-deer cull group was arrested for vandalizing deer traps in Kimberley. He later pled guilty to mischief.

In January 2016, I made a Facebook comment on a press release presented as an online news article about deer reportedly suffering in a deer trap in Cranbrook. I mistakenly said the lead spokesperson was a "convicted felon" for vandalizing deer traps and suggested he shouldn't be believed. (I later learned he was not technically convicted or a felon; he received a conditional discharge and the mischief charge he pled guilty to was not an indictable offence.) I apologized for my mistake. But ultimately, he sued me personally for defamation in the spring of 2016.

Initially, the lawsuit seemed frivolous and ridiculous to me. The rest of Invermere council and the Municipal Insurance Association of BC (MIABC) refused to provide defence coverage. The justification was because I was being sued personally and I didn't make the comments in a council meeting. This felt like a betrayal to me. In my mind it was clear: I was being sued because I was mayor and because of my involvement in the deer cull issue since 2011.

Since I had to pay for legal fees out of my own pocket, I made the mistake of hiring a young, inexperienced, and more affordable lawyer. The opposing legal council was a veteran litigator, and what seemed to me like a simple issue dragged on for over a year and eventually transformed into a complex seven-day civil trial with multiple witnesses and mind-boggling amounts of paperwork.

Within the first ten minutes sitting in the BC Supreme Court room, I knew that the judge disliked me. You could feel the disdain and impatience the trial judge had for my young lawyer. We didn't stand a chance.

PROVINCIAL RUN

I was trying to move up the political ladder from local government and jump into provincial politics. In the fall of 2016, I was successful in winning a nomination race for the BC NDP in the riding of Columbia River–Revelstoke. Well-liked incumbent MLA Norm Macdonald was retiring and endorsing me as his replacement. It was thought to be a fairly safe seat for the party.

But the excitement of winning the nomination only lasted a few days. The candidate who lost the nomination race, a former Invermere town councillor who is female and in a wheelchair, had complained to national media, asking how I met the BC NDP equity mandate—a policy that attempts to increase the diversity of candidates by limiting the options for men to run for the party in incumbent ridings unless they fit within certain minority or "equity-seeking" groups.

The party approved me as a candidate and said I could choose what I disclose and when. My local political advisors said I should stay quiet, not draw attention to my sexuality or to the equity mandate, and not directly engage with the opponent in the nomination race. Focus on the issues of the election, they said.

But when the losing candidate went onto CBC's *As It Happens* and many media outlets started circling asking questions about the equity mandate and my "mystery" fit within it, the senior people in the party switched. I needed to disclose immediately. A public non-answer was building this into a controversy. I suspected the losing candidate was hoping this would push the party to remove me as a candidate. One executive member of the party publicly outed me on Twitter without my consent.

From a young age, I was aware how pale and pasty I was. Some classmates were sure to remind me, saying things like, "You don't even need to dress up for Halloween. You already look like a dead person." At the age of about 7, my parents told me my uncle was going to move to China (actually Hong Kong). I asked if he was going to marry "one of those beautiful ladies from China." I don't know if it is some shame or dislike of how white and pasty I am, some genetic push for having children less pale than me, some push against the norm of a growing up in a very "white town" or a just a fetish, but for as long as I can remember, darker skin tones, darker hair colours, and "exotic" non-white people have been attractive to me, to the point that I found people with the same pasty skin tone as me to be unattractive, almost repulsive from a romantic or sexual sense.

My attraction to dark-skinned people existed long before I had any sense or understanding of white privilege or the challenges that BIPOC people face in our society. This attraction isn't exclusive to females; some trans women, cross-dressing men, and gender fluid people are attractive to me, and there have been some past encounters, but I have only ever been in heterosexual relationships.

I told the party leadership that I identify as bisexual, but that this was not publicly known. I don't know if the term fits perfectly. It's not a label that I feel super comfortable with and is not a large part of my life or part of my public identity. And now I was being pushed into making this public. I didn't have time, or even know how, to talk to friends and family. I called a local newspaper reporter; my biggest secret was now making headlines. It was messy, it was rushed, and it wasn't on my terms.

The whole situation hurt my credibility. Some people thought I was lying. Other people felt uncomfortable. They didn't know why my sexuality needed to be so public. And lots of people had just learned of the equity mandate and they thought the policy was stupid. It made them angry and dislike the NDP.

Politically, personally, locally, it was lose-lose. There was no point in trying to explain the nuances; there was no ability to debate the equity mandate. It was a gift to the BC Liberal candidate.

MAY 2017

In the same week, I lost the defamation trial and the provincial election, which I thought I was going to win. Both losses were crushing. The trial judge, who had previously donated to the BC Liberals when he was a lawyer, managed to have a 54-page judgement released in less than two weeks after the trial ended, days before the 2017 BC provincial election. The judge awarded $75,000 in damages, plus special costs. Part of his justification for the level of damages was because my words as mayor "carry more weight."

The opposing side was gunning for special costs of hundreds of thousands of dollars. During the discovery period prior to the trial, most of the attention was focused on my assets (basically, was I worth suing?). Post judgement, they immediately registered the judgement against my personally owned properties, and they were aggressive on opposing any refinancing. There were suggestions that they would try to push for court-ordered sales of my properties.

I chose to spend my 20s building assets and being involved in local government. I knew that I was giving up on fun, travel, and other life experiences. I had worked over 80 hours a week for years, staying up all night making gelato, spending lonely winter nights working the café by myself to save on labour costs. To lose all or most of my properties, properties I knew I could never get back, time that I knew I could never get back, felt like they were trying to take my youth, take the products of my hard work and smart decisions in my 20s and early 30s and wipe it all away, making it all a waste.

Realistically, if I had not assets, if I wasn't mayor, if I wasn't trying to move up into provincial politics, I highly doubt I would have been sued.

I had sold my business, my main income source, my first baby, Gerry's Gelati and Stolen Church Coffee Co. at the end of December 2016 so that I would be able to hit the ground running as MLA. In April, during the election and defamation trial, my wife and I found out that we were having a second child, and with that news, our beloved dog Piper almost died and needed emergency surgery. Thankfully, Piper survived the surgery and lived for several more years (which is why our daughter is named Veronica not Piper).

By early May 2017, I had no job, a pile of debt, a pile of legal bills, a huge judgement registered against my properties, and a new baby on the way.

There was a job fair at Kicking Horse Coffee. I showed up with a quickly printed résumé and before I could hand it in, I burst into tears. After several days of grieving, I signed up for the real estate course. I made gelato part-time for the people who bought my business, started serving tables at my friend's restaurant, and made and sold spicy non-alcoholic ginger beer at the farmers' market.

The stress and pain of the losses, the financial consequences, the shattering of ego, it took considerable time to heal. I couldn't fully shake the feeling that I had been screwed over. It's a helpless feeling. I pushed it away and tried not to dwell on it, tried not to become a bitter person because of it. This would have been a logical or understandable time for a mental breakdown, or a deep depression. But I had responsibilities and I had to fight to keep what I had worked for.

I started as a realtor in February 2018. The first few months were hard, the sales did not come immediately, and I still had the financial pressure of the lawsuit looming over me. But on a sunny warm day in May, I had three conditional deals come together on the same day, and from that point forward, it got easier.

One of the best personal and career decisions I ever made was in the fall of 2018, when I decided not to run again for mayor. It was becoming more difficult to be a realtor and mayor, both from a time commitment point of view, but also with potential conflicts of interest, especially with rezoning applications at the RDEK board. And I also decided that when people first heard my name, I wanted them to think "realtor" not "mayor"; however, I wasn't ready to quit Invermere Council cold turkey. I still cared deeply about the issues and the organization, so I decided to actively seek a demotion and run for council instead of mayor.

I eventually became one of the top agents in the Invermere/Columbia Valley area and one of the top-producing agents in the Royal LePage franchise system (as a single agent, not part of a team). I was doing over 100 transactions a year. The workload as a top-producing agent was intense—emails and phone calls all of the time, showing property evenings/weekends—and I was doing all of my own photos, videos, social media. Often, I would get overwhelmed and fall behind on the administrative paperwork.

AUGUST 2023

For a long time, the negotiations, the fast pace, the money—it was fun. But after years of running and grinding, it felt like things were getting gradually harder. The market was slowing, some listings weren't selling, and the properties that were selling were more complicated deals. Buyers and sellers all seemed to be on edge. And some of the people I was dealing with, they seemed to drain me of energy, they were so demanding. It was becoming less fun. I felt more and more guilt for missing dinners with my family and not spending time with my kids, for not trying to improve the relationship with my wife.

I knew that deep down my wife and I loved each other, but we didn't do a very good job of demonstrating that love to each other. Although we agreed on most parenting decisions, and we didn't yell or fight very often, we slept in separate beds and rarely had meaningful conversations. I practised a fair bit of avoidance. Neither of us seemed willing to try to reopen communication or rebuild connection with the other.

The relationship wasn't stressful. In a sense, it was comfortable (even boring), but the lack of connection, that lack of awesome, it was a weight. I had shame and guilt for not having a better, more perfect relationship. But even more so, I had shame and guilt for not knowing how to improve it—or not being willing to put in the time/effort or take the risk to try..

In addition to being super busy in real estate sales, I was doing a rural land development, and then trying to take the money from that land development and spin that into a renovation of a commercial building in downtown Invermere that I had just purchased. But in the spring of 2023, the second phase of my land development hit some delays, which I believe were bureaucratic and unnecessary, and the renovations were becoming far more complicated and expensive than I expected (because of building code issues and engineering issues).

Having spent almost my entire adult life as an elected official passing various policies and regulations, the irony was not lost on me when I had issues with trying to navigate approval processes as a developer or dealing with frustrating building code/engineering requirements on the commercial retrofit. A few key people in certain positions have a lot of power over interpretation of various policies and bylaws, and the timing of processing applications and granting approvals. And sometimes, the rules and procedures that staff need to enforce aren't great policy and don't make sense.

More and more local governments seem to require professionals' (like engineers) stamps on everything, and often it feels like these professionals, out of caution and a desire for more work, overdesign and over complicate things—and almost always recommend more studies.

When the interpretations of rules change mid-stream, it can feel personal. A bureaucrat with some vague policy to interpret and enforce can make someone's life miserable, and their project more difficult and expensive, if they want to. Or they can simply sit on a file for a while. It felt like that was happening to me, and when I tried to complain to elected officials and to senior managers with the regional district, it felt like it was falling on deaf ears. The issue was very technical and any kind of potential variance or review process would take months—if not longer. There was no quick workaround. It felt like no one was listening and no one cared.

By the end of August 2023, cash was tight. This feeling of being tight financially and having a lot of debt wasn't a new feeling; but with a lot of money coming in over the last few years, it was something I thought I had grown out of, something I didn't think I would feel again. But here I was once more; credit cards maxed out, renovation bills piling up, and cash disappearing fast.

I had just hired a second part-time assistant, but I wasn't good at delegating and I didn't have great systems in place. I wasn't using either assistant effectively. Some days it felt like they were adding more stress, not actually reducing my workload.

For at least the last year, I had been trying to get some solace from a light study of Stoicism and from Stoic quotes. During the summer of 2023, I got some posters printed with Stoic and motivational quotes. I was looking for purpose, I was looking for perspective, and I was looking for motivation. Looking back on it now, maybe this was a warning sign.

THE BOAT

My parents were never into boating or lake activities, and for almost my entire life, I told myself that enjoying the lake and having a boat was for "rich Calgarians," not for me. And for many years running the gelato shop, there really was no time in the summers for lake activities.

But, over time, more and more of my friends had got boats, and I knew more and more clients with lake access properties and boats. I felt like a fraud trying to sell lake-access properties and talking to people that were into boating when I never went myself. I wanted to spend time with my kids and give them experiences and opportunities that I never had. I didn't want to rely on friends inviting me onto their boat. I wanted the freedom and flexibility to go when I wanted to.

We had a really nice day trip with another family to Premier Lake. The kids were playing in the water and the sun was shining. Tied up at the dock was a beautiful little pontoon boat. It looked fairly new. I didn't need a fast boat. I wanted something social and relaxing. And that boat was perfect!

I started researching small, used pontoon boats for sale. Everyone I talked to told me to wait until next year, don't buy one this summer, the economy is going to get worse, prices will come down, just wait. But I couldn't wait; this felt important. I had been delaying gratification and doing things for the future my entire life. I wanted to indulge and enjoy things now. I wanted time with my kids now. But I wanted the time to be enjoyable to all of us. I couldn't enjoy watching them play video games. I hoped that being on the pontoon boat and around water would be something we could all enjoy.

I gave up on getting a used boat. The prices were high, and I didn't know anything about boats. I had enough old junk and things that needed to be fixed, and too many times in the past

The Safe Word is PINEAPPLE!

I had bought cheap stuff and regretted it later. I also had very little cash. I decided that buying a new boat and financing it was the only option. Through the process, I discovered my credit had been compromised, so it took extra paperwork to get the financing done. Nothing was simple or easy.

I was dealing with some difficult clients on a delicate deal, and there seemed to be so many urgent deadlines and things I had to do. I was supposed to pick up the new boat in Salmon Arm the next day. Instead of leaving Invermere that morning and having a relaxing travel day to Salmon Arm, it was now almost dinner time.

My wife, who was never that keen on buying the boat, was mad at how late in the day we were leaving Invermere. She said, "You are always late and always behind, and always doing what you want to do. Why are you even buying this stupid boat?" She wanted me to cancel the trip and cancel buying the boat. The kids picked up on her mood and piled on. Everyone was mad at me. It felt like the world was trying to stop me from getting the boat.

But I was determined. To me, the boat was symbolic of a life I wanted. I wanted to have time to float around on the lake, drinking beer and enjoying friends, family, and sunshine. I would go pick up the boat by myself if I had to. I would use the stupid thing myself if no one wanted to go with me.

My wife and kids ended up coming on the trip to pick it up. All along the way, there were phone calls and difficult people, deals hanging in the balance. But I was keeping the balls in the air, just barely.

THE ONLINE ATTACK

Around midnight, on September 1st, right before bed, I checked Facebook on my phone, and a post on a local passive aggressive Facebook group "Cheers & Jeers Invermere" caught my eye.

"Can people please explain to me how it is OK that local council members be buying up property in Invermere and still being allowed to be part of the board? Inquiring minds want to know. Is it just me, or is this not a conflict of interest? Some may think that I'm starting to stir the pot a little, however, just does not seem OK to me!!"

The post was written by a local lady who I only vaguely knew. It was already getting some comments and some traction—people were engaged. But who was she commenting on and what was this conflict of interest that she knew about?

The post was targeting either the current mayor of Invermere, who is in business and has some real estate holdings, or it was about me. The comments mentioned being in real estate. It was clear: It was directed at me. I thought engaging directly and talking in facts might help to clear up any misunderstanding, or at least slow down the vague attacks. I posted: "... I don't know if this is some kind of reference to me? Through a company I have recently purchased a commercial building downtown (old Lordco, or as I am calling it now 'O'Lord'). There was a patio application that went to council, I removed myself from any of the discussion or vote on that application." I also included a link to the encroachment application for the placement of a patio in road right of way.

The poster began to unload, saying, "You are buying up the town," "controlling shit," "you need to be called out." She suggested that I was personally benefiting from being on town council, that I needed to resign.

I was shaking. The words stung. Her comments were vicious; they seemed to come out of nowhere. Even though I knew her comments were bullshit, they still hurt, they still triggered me.

With it being close to 1 a.m., I suspected that the poster might be intoxicated. Maybe she would wake up the next morning full of regret? I responded, as calmly as I could, and resisted the urge to lash out. "I'm willing to have a civil discussion with people over facts, but unfortunately, I think this has gone pretty dark and pretty hostile pretty fast. I have nothing to hide and am happy to talk with anyone in person who has concerns."

The poster responded: "I am the mother of three boys and if any of my children go down the road that you have in politics and real estate I would be devastated as a mother that my kids have done what you do in our community!! And us having a civil conversation is never going to let people know the stuff you are doing and getting away with." She then went on to make reference to how disgusting it is to be bisexual and devolved into a homophobic rant that I failed to capture a screen shot of, and luckily do not remember very clearly.

The memories of the NDP nomination and the deer cull lawsuit came back. To dedicate over 20 years of my life to public service; to almost go bankrupt because of being involved in politics and the lawsuit; to rebuild and recover, to put my money where my mouth is, and invest in the downtown core because I wanted to do the right thing and encourage small businesses and local vibrancy; to believe my intentions were pure, and to have someone think so differently, perceive me as being or doing bad—it was devastating. It hurt to be so misunderstood, to be so unfairly judged.

But it also scared me.

The idea that somehow being on town council had got me some special treatment or allowed me to buy certain property—this fits a narrative that is popular right now. The story of some secret handshakes or special influence, the simplification of perceived success because of some shady dealings or conspiracy—that story is easy for people to embrace, especially if they don't know the people involved personally, if they are envious, if this is how they view the world, or if they are struggling with unfairness and trauma in their own life.

Despite this trigger, despite this attack on my credibility, this blow to my ego, rationally, I knew that the poster was suffering.

This was not the time and place to involve a lawyer; I would never wish that experience on anyone. I asked the group moderator to delete the post. I sent a message to the poster's boss, who I know, to express concern for the poster. Maybe she needed some help. I didn't want the poster to be fired and I wasn't looking to get anyone in trouble, but I was open to a face to face meeting if that would help. The poster's boss was apologetic and said she would look into counselling options for her employee. About two weeks later I bumped into the poster outside the Invermere liquor store, we were both caught off guard. She muttered under her breath, "Piece of shit." I kept walking and didn't engage.

CHAPTER 3
The Week of UBCM

SUNDAY, SEPTEMBER 17TH, TRAVELLING TO VANCOUVER

Always late for everything, I thought I had lots of time to drive to the airport in Calgary, Alberta, but with the traffic and the driving time, I barely made it to the airport with very little time to spare. But it was a beautiful drive. I listened to music, I relaxed. At the airport, security was a breeze. Almost missing a flight was a bit stressful, but not really a big deal. It didn't really matter that much, this was a relaxed travel day.

For the first time in my life, I took an upgrade to business class because it was only an extra $69. Flying business class was amazing. There is so much leg room, they feed you drinks, and they give you this cute little box of snacks. I don't know if there is a limit on the number of free drinks, but I got two gin and tonics on the flight to Vancouver. I did feel a bit guilty being in business class. I wished that all the seats in the airplane were like this. I wished there wasn't a curtain between us and the rest of the plane.

Landing in Vancouver in the early afternoon, I decided to indulge. When you are busy working and making money all the time, you don't really have time to waste at a casino losing money, but here was a rare opportunity. I got off the SkyTrain at the River Rock Casino and played some blackjack and a bit of slots. After buying two or three beers and some Asian noodle soup, and gambling for a few hours, I walked out of the casino up about $200. Not bad for wasting a couple of hours and having fun. Either my blackjack skills were improving, or I just got lucky.

Walking from the SkyTrain station to the Pacific Rim Hotel, I had to squint a bit and focus on which way to go. Was my eyesight getting worse or was I having a hard time concentrating?

Staying at the beautiful and luxurious Fairmont Pacific Rim hotel had become an Invermere tradition, going to back to when I was Mayor and the hotel first opened. Because the Convention hotel room block makes the nightly rate similar for almost all of the hotels near the convention centre, I could justify and enjoy the luxury, without much guilt.

During the evening of Sunday, September 17th, and most of the day of the following Monday, I spent a lot of time in the beautiful hotel room trying to catch up on and organize work, relax, and get ready for a crazy week. I was happy and comfortable, vaping some marijuana and sipping some hoppy beer.

The real estate market was shifting and slowing, deals were more complicated than before, and clients needed more hand holding. I had some guilt that I didn't always have time to nurture some clients because there were so many pressing deadlines, so many disclosure forms and Fintrac forms to fill out. Unfortunately, my newer part-time assistant was going to visit family in Ontario this same week. It was terrible timing. This was the week when I really could have used her help and relied on her more. I knew her absence would make these pressing deals harder and life harder, but I would do my best to keep the balls in the air and still have a

The Safe Word is PINEAPPLE!

super fun week participating in the Union of BC Municipalities (UBCM) Convention.

WEDNESDAY, SEPTEMBER 20TH, #1MILLIONMARCH4CHILDREN IN VANCOUVER

On the way back to the hotel from the convention centre, during the afternoon of September 20th, Councillor Pickleball (he was later given this name because the local pickleballers always called him first) and I stumbled upon quite the scene. A big parade/protest was going right by our hotel. We got closer, and slowly we figured it out: This was the counter protest to the #1MillionMarch4Children (people who were protesting over sex-ed curriculum and LGBTQIA2S+ rights in schools).

We watched the LGBTQIA2S+ folks doing what they love to do: a parade. They looked pretty damn happy and proud. We followed the crowd over to Jack Poole Plaza and saw the main protest, angry people yelling angry things, people claiming their only interest was to protect their children, but really angry about it and really angry about trans people. There was a chant. The angry people were yelling something like "Protect our children!" Both sides were beating on drums. And the other more fun and happier crowd was yelling back: "Trans rights are human rights."

But the beat was the same. It went back and forth for a bit. I realized that really, the two groups were effectively singing to each other. If it wasn't so polarized and with so much anger, from a distance, it would almost seem beautiful. Why were the sides so polarized? Why was there so much hate?

The day before, I got into a Facebook argument with a long-time local. I don't even remember what we were arguing about, because it was stupid. I caught myself. I tried to apologize and joked that I hadn't had enough coffee yet. We kind of made peace with each other. It was so tempting to take a side and start a fight, and it took effort and thought to realize just how dumb the argument was. I wanted to be on good terms with this guy. We could have different opinions but that didn't mean we were on "different sides." We didn't have to hate each other.

In that moment, with the chanting going back and forth, as the drum beats and rally calls rang through my ears, it really felt like an outside power was encouraging everyone to pick a side and pushing people to splinter into camps, to not look for shared values. It often feels like that pressure to divide is being amplified, like the screaming voice of hate on the megaphone in the plaza, through social media algorithms, fake news, and increasing mistrust of mainstream media and governments. We all seem to be on edge, pushed to not trust our community, to not trust our neighbours, to lead with fear and anger.

ON LGBTQIA2S+ PEOPLES AND SOCIETY

I definitely lean towards one side on this issue: I'm sexually attracted to some trans and gender fluid people. I wonder if other people have a secret attraction, and maybe this scares them and they lash out with hate. Of course, trans rights are human rights.

The #1MillionMarch4Children seemed to be suggesting that teachers were trying to groom children for pedophiles by teaching LGBTQIA2S+-inclusive curriculum. In my opinion, that is bonkers. None of my children's teachers and I think anyone in the education system is trying to do this; even if someone was, if school curriculum was so powerful and influencing, I would be able to speak French by now.

However, the left wing and those concerned with diversity and acceptance can take things too far. The fuss and offence some people take over being accidentally misgendered can be over the top. Some of the language and policies of large bureaucracies can become doublespeak nonsense. I am not sure that reverse discrimination, like the BC NDP equity mandate, is the answer.

Being too extreme, being too strict on mandating "inclusion," can actually go full circle and become alienating and illogical. It can give right-wing extremists ammunition in culture wars. Most people aren't extremists, most people aren't racists or homophobic, but average people can be made to feel that they aren't inclusive enough. It shouldn't be a contest. There needs to be room for mistakes, for blunt, honest language (even if that could trigger some people), for learning, for trying to be better.

Realistically, the percentage of trans and gender fluid people in our society is a very small number. Who really cares what gender someone else identifies as? Why is this such a hot-button issue? It really feels like this issue is being pushed as a wedge issue, a dog whistle, and something useful in dividing people. I saw a post online that asked, "Is it about dicks or about clicks?"

People are literally dying in the streets, have no housing. People are overdosing at record rates. Mental health and happiness are declining while anxiety is increasing. Things seem to be getting much worse very quickly. And yet, instead of focusing on solutions to problems we know are real, we spend our time and energy fighting about people's genitalia and their chosen pronouns? That is crazy!

EVENING, WEDNESDAY, SEPTEMBER 20TH, CUPE RECEPTION

One of my best friends from high school is named Greg. Greg is definitely a unique character, and we have a unique friendship. We can not talk for a year or two, and then I can announce that I am in Vancouver that day and we'll meet up for beer and catch up like we saw each other last week. Greg hasn't lived in Invermere since we graduated high school in 2000. His family moved away within a year of graduating, so he has no real pull to the area. The last time he went back was for our 10-year high school reunion in 2010.

For many years, I have invited Greg as a total non-UBCM person to crash various wine and cheese receptions. Many, many years ago, when I was still a councillor and before being mayor (maybe 2007?), there was a reception at the Vancouver Aquarium. We both went crazy with drinks, later ending up at the Roxy. I missed a 9 a.m. meeting with then -Premier Gordon Campbell the next morning. Roughly 8 years later, after many glasses of wine, Greg had a passionate one-on-one chat with then -Premier John Horgan.

I invited Greg and his new wife to the 2023 CUPE reception, the best party of the week. I skipped the earlier receptions, sipping a beer and vaping a bit of marijuana and trying to sort through emails and the work that was piling up. When I arrived at the reception, the room was fairly quiet; the lineup for drinks was short. I felt very chill and relaxed. But I realized something: For the first time in my life, I had no desire to move up politically anymore. I wasn't trying to meet anyone or impress anyone.

I was looking for deeper, real conversations, trying to figure out some solutions, trying to achieve something. I wanted to try to solve some problems. But most of the other people weren't there for deep conversation or problem-solving. They were working the room, looking for quick small talk, trying get food and drinks before the lineups got too long . . . I used to be that person.

Greg arrived and began double fisting glasses of red wine. Some of the staff and council members from Invermere vaguely knew Greg. He was a random but welcome addition to a fun night and a fun group of people.

The Safe Word is PINEAPPLE!

Many of us ended up at the Roxy later that evening. The live band was covering 90s and early 2000s rock. We all felt young and amazing! I was drinking and I was having fun, but I wasn't pounding drinks. Years earlier, there would have been a lot of tequila shots and I would have been looking for a one-night stand. I was in the moment with a random group of elected officials and some staff—people from across the province, partying it up in the big city. I felt content, happy. It was a great night. And my friend Greg was probably the drunkest of us all.

There was an elected official from a small West Kootenay town. I had talked with her a bit before and objectively I think she has a pretty face, but something about her energy had me wanting to talk to her more. I wanted to get to know her better. I chatted with her at the Roxy and established that she was happily married, learned about some of the story of why she moved to her small town and ended up running for town council. Near the end of that night, around 2:30 a.m., outside the club, a homeless lady commented on how nice her bracelet was. She chatted with the lady for a while and took the bracelet off and gave it to the now very happy homeless lady.

I told my new elected official friend: "I fucking love you," and I really meant it, but in a platonic way. Although I had only recently met her, I could sense how kind and genuine she was. But it is a weird thing to say, maybe even a creepy thing to say. Things were rushed, my group was leaving, there was a cab there, they were waiting for me, so I jumped into the cab and left the scene.

The next day, during UBCM events, I apologized to her for saying "I fucking love you"; however, it turns out that I didn't actually say it, I was just about to say it. My apology ended up being me telling her what I wanted to say the night before. She didn't seem to really care or judge me. If there were more people with her energy, her compassion, and her lack of judgement, I believe that all of our communities would be in a better place.

Gerry Taft

THURSDAY, SEPTEMBER 21ST, UBCM CONVENTION IN VANCOUVER

Resolutions were being debated on the floor at UBCM. Invermere council sponsored a resolution encouraging the province to soften the rent rate control rules for small-scale landlords. Landlords have limited opportunities to cover increasing costs, and as tenant rights and rent control protections get stronger, more and more small-scale landlords are selling units and those units are leaving the pool of available rentals forever. The Invermere resolution suggested a multi-pronged approach to retaining rental units, which could include subsidies, tax incentives, or allowing larger annual rent rate increases (currently, the province allows 3.5% each year).

I thought it would be a controversial resolution that would stimulate some interesting discussion and then narrowly pass or fail. When I spoke to the resolution, I disclosed that I was a landlord, a realtor, as well as an elected official.

The young urban elected officials pounced. What I heard was that all people who own investment properties are rich and privileged and they should have no rights, property ownership is effectively evil. "Market rents" is a dirty phrase that should not even be part of the conversation. And some of the older crowd, backing the resolution, talked about the horror stories of tenants and how terrible tenants are and how landlords have no rights.

In a crushing moment, an elected official from an urban Lower Mainland city, wearing a mask, stood up and tried to call a point of order, suggesting that because I was a landlord, this was a conflict of interest and that this resolution was for my own personal benefit. The resolutions chair was clear: This resolution was endorsed by Invermere council. It wasn't MY resolution.

Like the September 1st online attack, I felt misunderstood, that my motivations for this resolution were misunderstood. I was trying to find realistic solutions, but instead, I was perceived as being a greedy asshole operating out of self-interest.

The resolution was soundly defeated. It wasn't even close.

By speaking to the resolution, I likely hurt the policy concept. That is an unfortunate reality for our times; often who is saying something (and what you think about them or their identity) can have more of an impact on your opinion than the merits of the actual concept.

Although there were no specific hot-button debates or big headline-worthy arguments at the 2023 convention, it felt like there was more polarization, more frustration, and more fear.

I believe that deep down many of us, whether community leaders, engaged citizens, or just regular people, fear that things are getting worse, not better (and at a very fast pace). There is genuine frustration over not knowing how to solve the complex and interconnected problems our society faces, such as housing affordability, toxic drug overdoses, mental health crisis, and dramatic increases in homelessness. This fear and frustration seems to push some people to an extreme, to a simplified solution, to "pick a side" and embrace polarization.

EVENING, THURSDAY, SEPTEMBER 21ST, VANCOUVER, UBCM CONVENTION

I was working as the buyer's agent for some folks who wanted to buy a recreational condo in Radium Hot Springs. The buyers were very analytical, and it had been a struggle, but we had slowly come to an agreement on a selling price for the condo, but we were getting bogged down on dates on the contract and getting things signed by the deadlines.

The listing agent knew I was away, and it felt like he was making tight deadlines on the offer just to make everyone's life more difficult. Every change of a date or response from the sellers prompted the buyers to request a conference call with me and go into a detailed analysis. The timing wasn't lining up, things weren't flowing easily. And now this negotiation was going to spill into another day instead of being wrapped up that evening. Deep down, I suspected that my buyers would end up killing the deal over uncertainties in the strata. The whole thing felt like such a waste of time and energy, and I didn't feel like I had much time or energy to spare.

I joined Invermere council and then Invermere chief administrative officer (CAO) for a pleasant, casual dinner with drinks at a pub near the hotel. We had an intimate and fun dinner telling stories and getting to know each other a bit better. The CAO told a hilarious story about a squirrel that kept reappearing. We also jokingly "decided" that one of the councillors in Invermere should be the only point of contact for the aggressive local pickleball lobby group, crowning him as "Councillor Pickleball."

One of the things we commented on and laughed about was how the cleaning staff at the Fairmont Pacific Rim were very determined to rearrange toiletries. I noticed, for example, that they moved my marijuana vape pen every day. Other people commented on how their toothbrush and other items were always moved around. The afternoon turn-down service was very persistent; they were very determined to get into the room. Several times, I was in my room in the afternoon trying to send a few emails, and when I attempted to decline the turn-down service two staff members pretty much forced it on me (while being very polite). Later, in a paranoid moment, replaying the events of the week, I wondered if hotel staff could have been spiking my vape pen.

Another person attending the UBCM Convention—let's call her "Special Agent Button"—had a brilliant idea: We should crash the UBCM banquet and go have some more drinks. We arrived

The Safe Word is PINEAPPLE!

at the perfect time: dancing and drinks, everyone laughing. It was a great vibe.

Special Agent Button is a pretty funny and smart person, and I am not sure of all of her superpowers, but she was able to spot and connect with a fellow who was some kind of community relations person with a utility company. If you can find the right soft, friendly folks with company credit cards and follow them around, you can often score a round of drinks or a dinner. Although innocent enough when it is a utility company that doesn't provide service in your community and isn't really building market share, it has the potential to be a slippery slope, and you could see a situation where wining and dining could be taken too far. As elected officials, it's something to be very cautious about.

Special Agent Button had found her target. She said, "Let's follow this guy."

Let's call this guy "Bob." My memory was that Bob seemed kind of sober, and a bit bossy, but he said something like: "I am going to take you guys to a really expensive place, you are going to be really impressed."

I bumped into my new friend, the one I had professed my platonic love for, and she seemed willing to tag along on our adventures. Outside the convention centre, it was like magic: A super fancy Tesla Uber seemed to appear out of nowhere. I really wanted my new friend and her energy to be part of the rest of the night, but there weren't enough seats for her in the Uber—and she seemed kind of relieved to drop out. In a weird way, it almost felt like Bob didn't want her around, like she was excluded on purpose.

We piled into the Uber: our host Bob, me, Special Agent Button, and a friendly random guy from a small town north of Kamloops (also attending UBCM) who we had just met. We zipped over to Yaletown super fast.

Bob brought us into a nice-looking restaurant that was expecting us. We were the only table in the restaurant, and it was late.

Bob was excited to explain: "There is a champagne lounge in the back." Being from a small town, the term "champagne lounge" didn't mean anything to me. Bob was acting weird. He seemed very strangely determined to show off how much money he was spending on us. I would have been happy with one more beer. I didn't need to be impressed.

Bob ordered drinks for us; we didn't get to choose. I was sipping some kind of espresso/coffee/mocha cocktail, it tasted delicious, but it would not be something I would ever order. Being in this restaurant was so random, the situation was random. It was kind of funny, but it also felt kind of weird, like something wasn't quite right.

Suddenly, Bob pointed at me and demanded that I switch spaces with north-of-Kamloops guy. The demand was so socially awkward and so weird, and in that moment, Bob seemed volatile and strangely dangerous, although objectively, he wasn't a big guy and he didn't look particularly tough. I didn't want to follow his commands; however, I also didn't want to disobey him and make him angry. I decided to make it a joke and said to north-of-Kamloops guy, "Let's arm wrestle and see if we have to switch spots." I lost the arm wrestle on purpose (I was going to lose anyways). And then we switched spots.

Bob and Special Agent Button disappeared together for a few minutes.

I asked north-of-Kamloops guy how he knew Bob, and he said he didn't really, he just met him few days earlier at the conference and since Bob had been paying for everything, he just kept following him around. Bob returned to the table with Special Agent Button, and then he gestured for north-of-Kamloops guy to follow him, and they both left. With a moment alone with Special Agent Button, it felt important to have a serious conversation.

I leaned in. "Look, serious talk, zero judgement here, but this guy is spending a lot of money and he seems kind of weird. If you like him, that's fine. But please be careful. Don't piss this guy off or lead him on or embarrass him."

Bob returned without north-of-Kamloops guy. He went to pay the bill or talk to the server, and I joked to Special Agent Button: "Maybe he got that guy killed." At first, it was kind of funny, but then it wasn't really funny. It kind of felt like that could have actually happened—or at the very least he could have told north-of-Kamloops guy to leave, or had him kicked out.

Bob ordered us to leave the table and go to the champagne lounge. Bob led the way. As Special Agent Button and I were walking to the back room, I felt dread. Something wasn't right about the situation, something wasn't right about Bob. I was worried about Special Agent Button's safety. I was even worried about my own.

I grabbed Special Agent Button by her shoulders. Several days earlier, we had joked about a ridiculous pretend sexual joke, and the punchline was "The safe word is PINEAPPLE." In this moment, I said with so much intensity and so much seriousness: "THE SAFE WORD IS FUCKING *PINEAPPLE!* If either of us says it, we help the other one." I meant it with everything that was in me.

The champagne lounge was not very big, one long bar and some tables. Everything seemed to be black. The music was pounding, I think there was a DJ right there. No one was dancing, people were kind of swaying with the music. It looked expensive. All the other people in the club seemed to be wearing dark clothes. They were skinny, young, and emotionless. No one seemed to be laughing or smiling. North-of-Kamloops guy was in there, I was happy to see him alive. Like, legitimately happy he was still around. Safety in numbers.

There were three beautiful women, standing in a row, but they were fake beautiful: fake boobs, very done up, same black dresses, same hairstyle. They all looked equally blank, vacant. I didn't know what they were doing. I asked Special Agent Button, "Are they servers? Bottle services? Hookers? What do they do?"

She responded with: "I think they do whatever you want them to."

I didn't know the social protocols. How was I supposed to act? Should I stand at the bar or sit at a table? It was disorienting not knowing what I was supposed to do. We stood out. Us small-town folks, we didn't belong there. I wondered to myself, *Why did Bob bring us here? Who is Bob? What is this place? Has Bob been here before? Is he a regular?*

Secret Agent Button claimed that Bob knew everyone in the club and was talking to lots of people. I didn't see that. I was trying to figure out the place and how to act. We went out the back door for some reason. There were bouncers, there were limos lining the street.

I tried to subtly to ask a bouncer about Bob. "Does this guy come here often?"

Behind his tough face, the bouncer had a sparkle of humanity in his eyes, the first I had seen in a while. He seemed to almost feel bad for me, but he said, "I can't tell you anything."

Oh, great. A fucking secret place.

It felt so unsafe and so weird—evil actually. Was this some kind of evil gathering spot? Some secret elite cult-type thing?

We went back inside the club . . . and out of nowhere, Bob was stumbling drunk. He went from being bossy, maybe somewhat dangerous, to not being able to walk, messy, and stumbling around REALLY fast. He'd gotten drugged. It was the only thing that made any sense.

There was NO reaction from anyone else in the club. In a classy, expensive place like this creepy club, I figured it must be uncommon to be stumbling drunk or to be suddenly drugged. But from what I could tell, the people remained emotionless. There was no reaction. No one fucking cared, just one more secret.

The three of us small-town folks went from being afraid of Bob (I think I was the most afraid) to having to take care of him—an immediate pivot, an immediate role reversal. We got him out of the club and to a cab and sent him back to his wife and kids in Surrey.

After his cab drove away, I commented: "He has a wife and kids in Surrey? What just happened? Why are we here? This night can't get any weirder!"

But it did, at least for me.

Was he some kind of messenger, bringing us to this place for some reason? Or was he just an asshole trying to hook up? Did someone in the club drug him, or was he trying to drug one of us? Nothing made sense . . .

But now that Bob was gone and we were done with the club, I felt amazing. Like, really good. Everything was so funny, the danger had passed! As we walked by what appeared to be an escort getting in or getting out of a limo, I told her: "Invest in real estate," thinking that it was wise advice. She gave me a dirty look. She didn't want my advice, she didn't think I was wise, I was just a drunk asshole giving out unsolicited opinions.

As we wandered out of Yaletown, we stopped at a 7-Eleven. I bought some water and tried to make the others drink some. We started the walk back to the hotels near the convention centre. I was proud of myself for being so responsible and drinking water.

Along the way, I said, "I'm hungry, let's get some fast food." We settled on a Burger King on Granville Street. We were laughing at the concept of Burger King. I mean, who really goes there? It seems like such an unpopular fast-food franchise in Canada, you almost forget they exist. Around 3 a.m., we entered the 24-hour Burger King.

It looked like a war zone: a number of homeless people sleeping on benches and tables, security plexiglass between the employees and the customers, the bathrooms clearly locked, the door to the kitchen was even locked.

A friendly girl who was talking to herself recommended the gravy. Some of the other people in the lineup who looked homeless were friendly, too. We were really chatty and trying to make conversations with everyone. Objectively, it was probably a dangerous place to be, but it didn't feel dangerous at all. The staff wasn't friendly, but they weren't unfriendly. They were stoic, they were human, and there was no judgement. The shit that they must see . . .

One fellow was taking about four minutes to count out nickels to pay for his fountain pop. The girl at the till wasn't impatient, she wasn't judging. From what I could tell, she knew her job was terrible and she just accepted it. After finally getting his fountain pop, the guy tried to open the kitchen door. He knew it was locked, but he tried anyways.

There was a weird level of social protocol. The Burger King wasn't bothering with security or trying to clear people out—not at that time of day. They just let them be.

The gravy was fucking delicious. We ate in the restaurant and invited people to come sit with us, but nobody did. Maybe they thought we were weird. The food tasted really good, like really, really good. Although we were trying to be friendly, we didn't belong there. In a few minutes, we would be in our fancy taxpayer-funded hotel rooms. We were tourists visiting sketch town. We were laughing and having a good time, the other people weren't. The girl who recommended the gravy muttered something angry at us, or at me, on her way out. We probably deserved it. Later, I wondered if she maybe cast some kind of curse on me.

The class contrast was impossible to miss. I doubt anyone living outside of Vancouver has gone directly from the creepy champagne lounge in Yaletown to the Granville Burger King the way that we did, within 30 minutes of each other. To see the difference in wealth and society so dramatically and in such a personally experienced context—it shook me.

These two experiences gave me a very small taste of ultra wealth and urban poverty.

The Granville Street Burger King felt so much warmer, so much more human, so much more real to me. The people talking to themselves, shaking the door of the kitchen to open it, the workers dealing with whatever came—as crazy or unhinged as it might be, no one was pretending to be someone or something they weren't. There were no masks. No one was afraid to show their true emotions. Everyone was just trying to live and to survive.

If I had to pick between two worlds, I knew which world I would pick.

I knew in that moment, one of our biggest challenges in society is that we have such a hard time with contentment, with gratitude, with moderation, whether it's wealth or money, shopping, sex, drugs, alcohol, food, work, or trying to live forever. We have such a hard time with quality versus quantity. We have such a hard time admitting: "I have enough. I am full." We keep wanting more and more, we keep chasing. Almost all of us are addicts in one sense or another. Our society seems to feed on and be propelled by various addictions.

To keep chasing money as hard as I had been wasn't healthy. It wasn't going to make my family or my community better, it wasn't going to make me happier, it was pushing me closer to that creepy club and further from the real people in the Burger King.

What I saw at the creepy club with the unsmiling people, with the human flesh for sale to the highest bidder, with the drugs ending up in drinks, with the need for secrets, was that being ultra wealthy can be miserable, lonely, and cold. The people in that club seemed less human, less compassionate, and less authentic than the people struggling to survive at that Burger King.

Gerry Taft

FRIDAY, SEPTEMBER 22ND, UBCM CONVENTION

I only slept for an hour or two. Before going to sleep, I had been trying to write my thoughts down about the wealth gap and about the learnings from the creepy club and the Burger King. It felt profound, but I was struggling to articulate the feelings. I had a hard time focusing. When I woke up, I felt amazing, better than I expected to feel after such a short sleep and a night of drinking.

But as I stared at myself in the mirror, I couldn't decide if I should shave. It was really hard to make a decision. I texted a friend and asked them if I should shave. I had to really focus on showering and getting dressed. I was thinking about the events of the night before, trying to process what I had experienced, and small decisions and small tasks were very difficult to focus on. It felt like my head was in the clouds. Although I didn't really feel hung over from alcohol, I did feel kind of edgy, a little shaky, but good, energetic.

At the convention, I found my new friend, the one that narrowly missed being part of the night. I tried to tell her the story—it was so important for me to tell her—but I'm not sure I did a very good job of explaining it. I couldn't articulate properly why it was so profound to me, but I rambled on for over 20 minutes trying to explain it.

At the airport, I struggled to decide whether to check my suitcase. It was difficult to keep up with the pace of the security lineup. I ordered some food and a beer, and I tried to concentrate on the real estate contract for the Radium condo. It felt so strange. It was like the screen was blurry. I could not force my brain to focus on the contract details and the dates. It didn't seem important, but I knew it was. I tried to push myself to do the work, to focus, but I couldn't. I felt guilty that I couldn't. I promised myself I would do it when I landed in Calgary, I would do it later. All I

The Safe Word is PINEAPPLE!

wanted to do was talk. I wanted to call people and tell them about the night before.

Work suddenly felt overwhelming. I needed help. But instead of asking for help with this specific contract and clients, I sat in the airplane right before takeoff and texted another agent in my office to ask her if she wanted to set up a real estate team. It was a bold question and not something I had given a lot of thought to. It wasn't a terrible idea, but it was coming out of a sense of panic. It would take a lot of time and energy to figure that out and to implement it. I should have explored the idea a long time before. She responded that she was open to the idea.

During the flight, I had a wonderful conversation with the lady beside me. We talked about COVID, about society and class systems. We talked for the entire flight. Chatting took my mind off my anxiety and guilt around work.

When I got off the plane at the Calgary airport, I felt like a confused old man. I felt so tired, and it was difficult to concentrate on using the stupid app for the airport parking lot. The screen of my phone seemed blurry. I had to squint and use all my energy to focus and type my credit card info.

I phoned home and my son Kelvin answered. I told him that Daddy was really tired and I was going to stay the night in Calgary. I asked him if that was okay, and he said, "Sure, Daddy." I broke into tears. I hadn't talked to them much during the week, but I also felt so relieved. I knew I couldn't drive back to Invermere that evening.

Booking the hotel was difficult; navigating to the hotel was difficult. Everything was so complicated.

I finally made it to the hotel. At the front desk, there was a grumpy-looking, younger Indo-Canadian woman working. She would have seemed attractive to me if she hadn't been so obviously miserable. I had a sense that this hotel was still trying to appeal to families and regular people but because of the price point and location in Calgary, probably got a fair number of less family-oriented clientele.

I had no filter and said exactly what I was thinking: "Do you get a lot of hookers staying here?"

She didn't seem surprised or uncomfortable with the question. She just gave a really honest answer: "Well, once we find out, we kick them out, but yes, there are some that stay here for a while until we know."

She told me that there were some people who lived in the hotel, like the engineer in the oil patch who paid the full nightly rate and stayed for months at a time, coming and going from work up North. He kept the same room. This was his home. She told me she was a student. She had an exam she was worried about and she should be studying for.

After this weird five-minute conversation, when I left, she was smiling. She didn't look grumpy anymore. Someone had listened to her. Someone had a real conversation with her.

When I got to my room, it seemed like the room card worked, but the door was locked on the inside. I couldn't get it to open. Was it possible the front desk attendant had given me the wrong room card, or was someone already in the room? I'd probably distracted her while we were talking.

I went back down to the front desk. The Indo-Canadian woman was busy with another customer, but another young woman, a very good-looking fair-skinned girl, was available (although normally I don't find fair-skinned people overly attractive, this young woman could have been a model). I told her I couldn't get into my room. She reprogrammed the key and said she would come help me.

I tried to refuse. "That's not safe. You really shouldn't be alone with guys in a hotel like this. I mean, I'm safe . . . but . . ."

She gave me a weird look and started walking to the elevator. It turns out she was from the Ukraine and had only been in Canada for a few months. I was wondering why such a pretty girl was working at this hotel.

She got the door open with no problem at all. I felt so stupid. Then I thought it might make me look sketchy: I had just chatted up the other girl for five minutes and now I was getting this one to come to my room. I was so worried what people were thinking about me.

Suddenly, I had this strong feeling that I knew what I needed to do. I grabbed $100 from my wallet and gave it to her. She tried to refuse. I said, "I am sure you have seen some stuff. You need this more than I do," and I meant it. I closed the door.

But then I started thinking, *What if she tells the East Indian girl? The East Indian girl will be mad that I didn't tip her.* I had such a pile of work that I should have been doing, yet in the moment, I was so concerned about what the front desk staff thought about me, and about what was fair from a tipping perspective. So, I went back downstairs and casually slipped $20 on the counter near the Indo-Canadian girl. I figured that $20 was fair. I mean, she didn't help me with the door.

I tried to do work. I still didn't have any focus, and now another a deadline for responding to the counteroffer had passed. I couldn't fix the contract and send it for signing. Technically, the deal was dead. I would have to write a whole new contract and start over. I couldn't even think through those steps. I sent an email to my clients suggesting that we shouldn't work together anymore and how I thought they didn't even want to buy the condo and how the whole thing was pointless.

I cracked a beer and paced the room. I started dreaming up ways try to fix the problems of society. *Maybe UBCM could be a vehicle for change? Maybe UBCM needs a secret fraternity of long-time members who would be more effective at making change* than *the overall membership, they could work behind the scenes with the executive and senior staff, but wait—that's not a good idea because that is secret. There has to be more radical change, we have to deal with homelessness, what is being done isn't working, resolutions aren't working . . .*

I got a text message from my best friend, Justin, and another from a newer friend, Trevor. They are both great guys who are very grounded, have good morals but also get the current world. They push the envelope and grow in business, but they don't fuck people over. Getting those messages and having brief text conversations was exactly what I needed in the moment. It helped to ground me a bit and reminded me of the good of humanity. It made me feel loved, it helped take away guilt and shame. I could literally tell these guys anything about me, and there would be no judgement. In the moment, a super weird thought for me, but I knew these two, in that moment, were my little angels.

I was spinning, I was spinning hard, I paced and thought, I wrote speeches in my head. I was having fun, but I knew it wasn't healthy, I knew this wasn't good. I was definitely manic. I thought about my double life, how being an elected official and attending conferences was kind of like a secret affair, it was taking me away from my family and my main career. Maybe I was having a breakdown because I was realizing that I needed to break up with UBCM and with politics. Maybe it was time to grow up and admit that the relationship wasn't healthy. Maybe I could be more effective from the outside?

I had a sense: *You don't have enough time. There isn't enough time to try to work up the executive ranks. Things will be too far gone by then, and you need to do more important things with your life.*

I realized that I needed to write a book on saving UBCM and/or society, and talk about my experiences in Vancouver. There was something significant about that creepy club. I was right on the tip or the edge of a profound realization, to some amazing insights and solutions to all of the problems . . . but I couldn't focus enough to document them. The thoughts were jumping around, I had the answers, but I couldn't concentrate enough to document them.

As I spun more and more out of control, it shifted from being fun to being scary. I slept in one-hour increments. I started journalling and documenting times and thoughts, trying to keep a record every time I woke up. Something wasn't right about the situation. It felt like something or someone was gaining control of my thoughts. I had to document everything, leave a record.

CHAPTER 4
You Can't Cheat Death

EVENING, SUNDAY, SEPTEMBER 24TH

Several minutes earlier, I had said goodbye to my kids and was ready to die. In the moment when I could feel death coming, the fire alarm in the hospital had gone off. And now I was sure that someone or something was trying to kill me, or trick me into choosing death.

I continued to talk in the parking lot at the Invermere hospital, and my sister continued to film. First the battery on my phone died, and then I got my sister to film on her phone, but then the battery on her phone died. Technology was being really glitchy.

I was on edge. Part of me was so happy to be alive and to not feel like I was dying anymore, but part of me was scared. There was absolutely no way I was going back to my deathbed in the Invermere hospital, and I was feeling uncomfortable even being in the parking lot. We agreed that I shouldn't go home to my wife and kids. Instead, the interim plan was to spend the night at my mom's house.

Why did I feel like I was going to die? What, or who, was trying to kill me or make me choose to die?

My mom is fully and completely a conspiracy theory believer, or "freedom fighter" (I think she would prefer this title). She gets a lot of it from her sister (my aunty Cathy), who has always been into interesting things and going against the grain. Cathy and family were vegetarians in the 1980s, when it wasn't easy to be vegetarian in Calgary, Alberta. When it started to get easier in the early 90s, they started eating red meat. They have been through a lot of phases/fads/trends, and whatever Cathy and family are involved in, they go in with 110% commitment, and my mom usually follows, although generally with a bit less zeal.

COVID vaccines were a sensitive topic in my family, like many others. My sister was pretty leery and ended up traveling to the US to take Johnson & Johnson because she had to take something for her job. My mom is absolutely opposed and afraid of them, and she remains unvaccinated. The rest of us (I, my wife, Dad, and so on) took whatever we could get, without much thought.

Having been in local government politics since 2002, having a small taste of the bureaucracy and complications in dealing with the provincial and federal governments, it has always seemed impossible to me that a large-scale conspiracy could be pulled off by a government, especially anything involving the Government of Canada. They struggle to pay their employees; they seem completely incompetent at delivering services. How could they keep anything secret and be part of any master plan?

Whether it was vaccines or Justin Trudeau, there were things my mom and I just couldn't talk about anymore. It had unquestionably strained our relationship. But despite the differences of opinion, we agreed to disagree and still maintained a relationship.

But, at this point, nothing made sense anymore. I was willing to suspend all my beliefs and consider a wide range of perspectives, perspectives that I had previously dismissed. As I entered my mom's house, I decided that I needed to know more about what she believes in.

My mom explained that there are some elite people in positions of power who have been corrupted and who are pushing an evil agenda. *Okay, that could have an element of truth.*

She mentioned that they operate based on needing consent, but it is not informed consent, it can be a tricked, sneaky type of consent. *There does seem like there is some tricked or non-informed consent in the world right now.*

My mom continued, saying there is a headless beast, that the head has been cut off, and the evil agents are operating without a real plan. *Okay, maybe as a metaphor, but I'm not sure that literally is the case.*

Then it started to get very specific and very weird. There are "white-hat" people who are trying to do good things against the deep state. And there are pedophile rings. Hollywood and sci-fi movies are foreshadowing what is coming, and are a form of the tricked consent. There are lizard people. Many of the world leaders are not really humans; they are actors or alien lizards pretending to be humans.

These specific details still seemed ridiculous to me. I felt impatient, I still felt like time was slipping away, I didn't have a lot of concentration or patience for complicated details. Especially things that couldn't easily be proved or disproved. Every time my mom would go into weird specific details, I would say: "Too much detail, that doesn't really matter, move on." I kept trying to get her to focus on the high-level concepts, and she kept wanting to get into very complicated specifics. None of these weird specifics were helping me to understand my situation.

EARLY MORNING, MONDAY, SEPTEMBER 25TH

You were supposed to die yesterday. You can't avoid this. You need to decide. It wasn't really a voice, more a message. I didn't really see it or hear it, but I felt it. I was lying on my mom's couch (comfy enough to sit on, but not very comfortable to sleep on.) It was the early hours of Monday, September 25th. I had slept for an hour, maybe two.

The message continued. *The scales are tied: You are equally good and bad. Since it is a tie, you get to* choose *which side you want to be on.*

I was given a preview, a vision, kind of like a dream, but I think I was awake. There was a crowd of people, and I could see a white aura around some of the people, they had glowing white light in their eyes or sometimes their entire face. They were helping people, they had healing energy, they were doing good deeds. They felt so warm, so perfect. It was so peaceful.

And then it changed. Now some people had black circles where their eyes should be, they were doing bad things, pushing and tripping people, encouraging people to be angry, they felt cold and angry. They were greedy and selfish, and encouraging others to be the same.

The message returned: *You need to pick which side you want to join. And you are one of the last people to pick. There is going to be an ultimate war very soon between both sides, they are waiting for you to pick before the war can begin.*

I thought about the current situation. The people with the white eyes seemed to be good spirits, like little angels on earth, they seemed like a great side to be on. The people with the black eyes seemed to be evil spirits or little demons, clearly not the side anyone would choose to be on. But an ultimate war between both sides? That didn't sound good at all, that sounded like it would end humanity. It felt really scary and really wrong.

Something about the choice didn't seem right, like it was a trick question. If the scales were really tied, and I chose the "good side," that could be considered a very selfish choice. By making that choice, might I actually tip the scales and push myself over to the "bad side"?

I thought back to what my mom had said about tricked consent.

I was getting the impression that truly joining either of these sides meant it was some kind of afterlife, so it looked like this still involved dying. I really didn't want to die, I liked my life, I really just wanted my normal life back . . .

Why did there need to be an ultimate war? Couldn't there be some grey people, some people in the middle keeping the two sides from destroying each other? I thought about it. I shouldn't get to decide. If this was some kind of heaven or hell on earth, or ultimate judgement between good and evil, the decision should be based on my actions, not something I chose. I needed more time on Earth to prove myself one way or another. Basically, an overtime. I would try to do some good, I would make some commitments, I would try to be a better person, and then whatever or whoever was the judge could decide which side I belonged on, based on my actions.

I called a big "time out" or "point of order." The message back regarding my ask for more time seemed to say: *It will be considered.*

And then I was given more visions. I had the power to see who had white eyes or black eyes. I could basically see who was good or evil or being influenced by these forces. I got shown the faces of a few specific people, mostly work colleagues, I was shown that they had black eyes. It seemed to me that this was a warning: Watch out for these people.

I thought it would be pretty depressing and disappointing to see black eyes in different people, I didn't want to judge people. I would rather believe that all people are inherently good and trying their hardest, even if they occasionally do bad things. I would like to believe that there are very few evil people or people purposely doing bad things. So, I declined this power.

Next, I saw the world full of patterns and symbols. Everything made sense, strange situations seemed to have reasons behind them, there were little fairies and mystical things, there were mathematical formulas. Everything had a pattern and a reason. It seemed really cool, but it was a lot to absorb and understand—and I enjoyed my old life, I enjoyed the mystery. I didn't need to see or understand all of the patterns. I declined this power as well.

Next was a big door. I cracked it open only slightly. It was complete white light and ALL POWER. It was the ultimate everything, the power of God or a creator or something far beyond human. The feeling was so strong, just being near the cracked door was overwhelming, but I knew *I can't handle that shit*. I slammed the door shut.

My knowledge of world religions is not that deep, but I think I vaguely understand the concept of Christianity and the idea of a Second Coming, of a representative of God coming back to Earth to lead people in a time of need. I thought about the current world, about cult leaders. The last thing our world needs is another self-proclaimed demigod or messiah, another cult leader. And if there really was a person with divine power, they would definitely get locked up or killed. There would be a lot of forces out there that would not want this person to have any credibility.

If God, which I am not even sure if I believe in, was going to try to find a human to help the world, maybe "they" would pick a non-religious person, a flawed human, and maybe instead of leading people, this person could try to empower others. They wouldn't be worshiped, they would just help to connect with other "grey" middle people and help to build local capacity in communities. Help to push against corruption and broken, illogical systems, but to do it in a gentle and grassroots way.

Using my negotiating skills as a *realtor* and a politician, and borrowing heavily from the concepts and principles of the excellent keynote speech given by John Herdman at the UBCM convention (to paraphrase from what I remember of his speech: Instead of striving for perfection, strive for 80% or even 90%, focus on "good enough," focus on being honest with yourself, stop lying to yourself, have strong personal morals and boundaries. Redefine or redesign your life. Professional success is not sustainable if your home and personal life is a mess,) I set about writing a quasi contract to extend my life.

I opened my laptop and titled the document "The Source Code." As I typed, I felt that I did have immense power, this document would grant me special powers. It was like a computer code, whatever I typed in here was real and binding. This was the basis of my new life. A redesign. If what I asked for was reasonable and not too greedy, not too selfish, it could come true, it would be considered, and then I could get more time on Earth and I could help to make the world a better place. But if I was too greedy, too selfish, too evil—this could be the end.

I asked for:

- More time on Earth—either one more day, seven more days, or 41 more years. The greater power could decide what I deserve, but I couldn't live in fear of dying every single day if I survived the first week.
- It not to be a brain tumour.
- This to not be a situation where I was in a coma and dreaming all of this up, although if that was reality, I had no choice but to accept it.
- Me to be not too crazy, if I had to be crazy for the rest of my life. I'd be OK with just "crazy enough" (whatever that means.)

- Any kind of immediate "ultimate war" or major conflict involving Invermere to wait. I needed at least a month to get my mind settled and get used to being "reborn". I reserved the right to ask for more powers if things were really bad after October 31st, but until that time, this document was locked and no bad forces could access it and its power.
- My old life back. I wanted to raise my kids, I wanted to be able to do fun projects and contribute to making Invermere and BC a better place.
- Special powers, like a little more empathy and a little more intuition, and the ability to have a healthy relationship with alcohol (to stop drinking whenever I wanted to.)

In return, I would live my life based on this personal code of conduct:

- Family has to come before community; I needed to focus on my kids first.
- I will try not to lie to myself.
- I will try not to lie to others, but I accept that they may not always be ready for my full truth.
- I will ask for consent first. I will not force my views or ideas onto other people.
- I will never intentionally harm myself or anyone else, but I am not responsible for other people's feelings and triggers (offending someone is not necessarily harming them.)
- I will lead with love and compassion, not fear and anger.
- I will try to drop all shame and guilt.
- I will have faith in my neighbours and my community, but even if they fail me, my love for Invermere is unconditional.
- I will work on ideas to improve society and systems, but my focus is Invermere. I am not responsible for fixing

The Safe Word is PINEAPPLE!

everything, I cannot control the outcomes, I am not responsible for saving the world.
- I will put limits on how much I work and how much money I make.
- I will never be worshiped; I am a flawed human, not a god.
- I will have more fun!

In my head, I pictured a box, a sanity box. Within that box, I could be eccentric and weird, I could push up against societal norms, but if I ever crossed out of that box into something completely crazy, if I were ever in a situation that I absolutely could not handle or could not control, if I were ever going to violate the principles of my personal code of conduct, if it ever seemed hopeless, I would use the SAFE WORD. I would have faith that some kind of miracle or good spirit would help me, that my neighbours and community would have my back, that somehow the flawed systems wouldn't fuck me over. I would stop fighting and just accept the situation. If I yelled "PINEAPPLE," I would give in and give up. It was time to let go and have faith.

I had to protect the laptop. I also realized I had to be careful what I told and to whom. People were not necessarily going to believe me, and I might now be a target. I felt that there was going to be persecution—people and bad forces were going to try to discredit me or lock me up. I had to be very careful balancing in the grey and not picking between good and evil.

Shortly after writing the source code and negotiating to extend my life, I heard noises coming from my mom's bedroom upstairs. It was heavy breathing. Something wasn't right. There was a chance that my mom was dying. Maybe that was what this was all about, maybe it wasn't about me dying, maybe all of this was about my mom dying. But there was also something that didn't feel right. I had just been exposed to an incredible amount of information and power. I had this fear: What if some evil spirit had taken over my mom's body, and if I went upstairs to check on her, there would be some kind of battle?

I couldn't do this alone, either dealing with my mom dying or some battle with an evil force. I called my sister. It was about 4:30 a.m. My sister answered (it turns out she wasn't sleeping much that night and wasn't very surprised to get a call from me.) She agreed to come to my mom's house. When she arrived, we both started walking up the stairs to my mom's room, but I realized that I had forgotten the laptop in the living room. Maybe it was a trick to get me to go upstairs and distract me, and someone or something would take the laptop? I grabbed the laptop, and we went upstairs.

As we entered our mom's bedroom, she woke up. She had been slightly snoring. She was confused as to why we were both standing there.

I wanted to explain everything to my sister. I didn't want my mom to know too much. I felt like having coffee, so my sister drove us to the Invermere McDonald's. It was around 5:30 a.m. We sat in my sister's truck in the parking lot. We never got any coffee.

I mentioned my visions of white eyes and black eyes, the source code, the looming ultimate war, and that I somehow was an important piece of all of this. My sister was pretty calm and she listened. She didn't say much.

I felt some anxiety and paranoia about my kids and my immediate family. It occurred to me that if "they" couldn't get me to die, they might try to harm my kids in some way. I had to get home and protect my kids. Also, I might have only negotiated one more day on Earth, and if this was the case, I wanted to spend as much time as I could cuddling and being with my kids.

My sister drove me to my house and dropped me off around 6:30 a.m. My wife greeted me. Something was weird though. She was being so sweet, her voice was a bit higher. She was being really

The Safe Word is PINEAPPLE!

nice, almost too nice. It seemed kind of fake. I told her I wanted to cuddle with the kids.

My wife said, "They are in your bed, come to your bed." And she led me towards my bed. It looked so comfy and warm, but I had this sense: *This feels like a trick, like a deathbed.* I turned on the light; the kids were not in the bed.

My wife was very ANGRY with me for turning on the light. I saw her eyes, they were black ovals, she was a demon . . . she was being controlled by the bad side.

I ran to my son's room and turned on the light. Both kids were in bed together sleeping. I jumped into the bed and put my arms around them. My wife followed, she was very angry.

She said, "They have school. Why are you waking them up? Turn the light off."

There was something about the light, I thought. *The tricks are easier in the dark, the demon doesn't like the light.*

I remembered: There was no school that day. It was one of the many endless, unexplainable non-instructional days that happen all of the time. I said, "There is no school today."

The demon became very suspicious. I knew a lot more than I was supposed to know, I realized, I couldn't be too smart or things would intensify, things would really get dangerous. So I started to fake a bit, saying that I was confused and was not understanding what was happening. I couldn't let the demon get any more angry or suspicious.

But the crazier and more confused I acted, the more it became real. A wave of brain fog came in. It became a real struggle to jump between confused and rational. I started to feel like different sides were trying to control my brain. If I focused hard enough on one, it would win out, but when I switched to the other it would start to win.

To my surprise, my kids did not seem equal in that moment. My son Kelvin felt cold, indifferent, completely uncaring about me or the demon, he was neutral and not going to participate. But my daughter Veronica was so warm, she had some kind of positive power, a glow. She was the target of the anger from my demon wife. Veronica was the one at risk in that moment. She was the one that needed immediate protection.

We ended up downstairs in the kitchen and living room. The situation seemed so out of control, my mind was out of control. At one point I said the safe word, "PINEAPPLE!" Veronica started speaking kind of funny, not like a 5-year-old would. She looked at me sideways and spoke with her voice but with a message that seemed to come from beyond her: "Daddy, you don't need to use that word anymore, I will help you."

It felt in that moment that my daughter was being guided by the good forces.

My laptop was on the kitchen counter, and I realized that this was a real-life test. A test between family and community. Do I let the demon potentially hurt my daughter or do I let the demon and the bad side have access to the source code and what power could be contained within that laptop? Giving up that laptop in that moment meant giving up on Invermere. Meant choosing my child over Invermere. It was such a hard decision, but if it was the only option, protecting my daughter was the decision I had to make. I picked Veronica. I sat on the couch with her and put my arm around her.

I was considering many perspectives at the same time. My wife being a demon felt so real, but I knew it didn't really make sense. You hear of stories, people who hurt their loved ones and who are suffering from delusions. Maybe this was a delusion? Maybe someone or something was trying to make me think my wife was evil? Maybe I was being framed, they wanted to make it look like I am unsafe to be around my family.

I knew that I would never hurt my wife or my kids, I knew I had to protect my kids. But I had to prove this. I needed witnesses. I needed to consider all the options.

My wife, who still seemed like a demon but now a slightly less scary one, announced that she was going upstairs for a shower. This was my opportunity to protect Veronica and the source code, and find witnesses. Maybe I could do it all?

I casually slipped the laptop under my arm and Veronica under the other. I put my shoes on and ran out of my house down the quiet residential street. I had to have faith in community and in my neighbours. It was around 7 a.m., and I was yelling as I ran: "I will not harm anyone, I will not harm myself. WE are not safe. Someone please protect my daughter."

I was trying to wake people up and create a scene. I needed witnesses that I was not hurting my family, I was trying to protect them in the only way I knew how.

As I ran down the street, things seemed dreamlike. Was this real life? Maybe I really had died, and this was some kind of purgatory or afterlife? Or I was in a coma and imagining all this stuff? Or maybe this was really happening? I had to consider all of the options, but in the moment, I really didn't know which was real.

Some neighbours shunned me. They watched, or called the police, but they would not take Veronica, they were scared of me. My wife was behind me trying to grab Veronica, but I would not let Veronica go until a mutual friend and neighbour, who is an energy healer (and an all-round amazing person,) calmly stood at the front porch of her house and said, "I will keep Veronica safe."

I could trust her. She was the perfect person to help, it was a miracle! I thanked her, and I quickly walked away.

I wanted to bounce around town and protect the laptop and only deal with people who I knew and could trust. I needed to share how I had almost died, had negotiated an extension to my life, and now someone or something was after me.

The police would be looking for me. I had the sense, if I got locked up, *they* would get to me, I would get drugged up and shut up, maybe forever. I had to rely on my intuition to survive. If my heart started to pound, if I felt fear, it was a sign of danger—I should bounce. If I felt calm, then the person and situation was safe—at least for the moment.

A neighbour with a big diesel truck, who never waved and seemed unfriendly, was trying to smile at me. He was inviting me into his truck, strongly pushing me to go with him. He made me uncomfortable. At the same time, an East Indian woman on a bicycle was leaving a nearby townhouse. She had not been a witness to the scene of me running down the street with my daughter a few minutes earlier.

I quickly analyzed the situation. If there is some bigger conspiracy in or around Invermere trying to trap me, it was very unlikely that this woman would be part of it.

I wanted to talk with someone, I wanted to walk with someone. But my new code was to ask for consent. I asked if I could walk with her.

She said, "I am on the way to work, I work at A&W."

I said, "Oh, that's okay, you can ride your bike to work, and if you are okay, I will just walk beside you and talk for a bit, is that okay?"

She seemed to have a look on her face that was a mix of confusion and "I don't give a shit, I just need to get to work.".

I started walking and talking with her. I had sold a condo to her manager. The manager had been a tough client at first but over time, once trust was built, she and her husband proved to be really nice people.

After walking for a little, I realized one of my other new life codes was that I had to tell the truth to other people. I hadn't figured out tone yet, and I had no filter. I have a physical attraction for dark-skinned people. And in particular, I find many East

Indian women very attractive. It occurred to me that this was not a coincidence that I was walking beside an East Indian female. This was another test. Was I going to stay true to my new code and tell the truth?

I really wanted to keep walking and talking with this girl, and she wasn't really that attractive, at least not to me. But I had to tell her, but of course it was going to sound creepy and crazy, because it was a really weird thing to say to someone at 7:30 a.m. (or probably anytime of the day).

I was running four or five situations through my mind, including still not being sure if I was really alive or not. Thinking everything was potentially symbolic and a test, but also trying to be aware of social norms, and people's feelings, and trying to ask consent.

I told the young lady on the bike: "I need to tell you something weird," and then I blurted out: "I find East Indian women attractive but I don't really know that much about the culture, although I am sure the culture is beautiful, it just doesn't really interest me that much, and I don't really think you are attractive, so you don't have to be scared."

She looked concerned. I couldn't blame her. I had to ask for consent again. "If you are uncomfortable, I will stop walking with you?"

She said, "Ah . . . Yes, please."

"I understand, thank you for listening."

I crossed the street.

Now I was alone, definitely a target for someone evil or the police. But it occurred to me I was near the home of the folks who had bought my old business, Gerry's Gelati. They are pretty open and neutral people. If there was some big worldwide or townwide conspiracy of good versus bad, they would be more likely to be in the missing middle/grey category. I knocked on their door.

They answered and invited me in. They were concerned and knew that something wasn't right, but they were kind and let me talk for a while. I tried to gently open up about the conspiracy stuff, someone or something after me, the creepy club in Vancouver, but I got resistance, there was some pushback.

I knew, as soon as I got resistance, as soon as someone didn't want to hear the truth, my truth, they might be getting taken over by the evil forces, or at the very least, I had to pull back and not force my beliefs onto other people. I thought to myself that spreading my new message was a push and then a pullback. Don't force it onto people, introduce it and then seek consent before going any further. There was pushback. I felt uncomfortable being there any longer. I got out of there fast and bounced down the street.

And there was the police car, basically waiting for me. I sort of tried to run, but that wasn't going to work. The police officer looked kind of evil, he was definitely one of *them*. I was going to get locked up.

With no other choice, with the RCMP officer standing in front of me, I needed a miracle, I needed help. I firmly said, "PINEAPPLE!"

The RCMP officer's eyes were not black ovals, he was calm, and after I had said "PINEAPPLE" he cracked a bit of a smile, his face lit up a bit, he was probably trying not to laugh. He seemed human, he seemed real, he didn't seem evil anymore.

He gently guided me into the back of the police car, no cuffs. He left the door open for a minute.

I tried to rationalize with him. "I am not harming myself or anyone else."

He said, "But you are acting weird. We just want you to get checked out at the hospital."

I really had no choice, and he was being kind and gentle. I gave in. We drove to the hospital. I got sent back to the same room I had been in the day before, the room where I almost died.

Nothing had been touched. Sitting on the table was the unfinished Chinese food right beside my death bed.

I ran out of the room, going in the wrong direction to a dead end. The RCMP officer calmly followed me. I said, "I don't want to be here."

He responded, "Gerry, you are arrested under the Mental Health Act, you can't leave right now."

That hit me like a ton of bricks. Me . . . arrested under the Mental Health Act?? I never thought in my entire life that would ever happen to me.

"If I am not going to harm myself or harm anyone else, why am I arrested under the Mental Health Act?"

Again, the RCMP officer cracked a smile. In that moment, it felt like we were in a cheesy re-enactment, some kind of reality TV show or *Truman Show*–type thing. We were both playing parts. This officer wasn't a professional actor and he was having a hard time keeping a straight face. I liked seeing the humanity, it reminded me that he wasn't evil. Maybe this was a miracle, maybe a lot of the good people in town and good forces were working to protect me. I had to consider all options.

But then the battles in my brain took over. There were waves that were so strong. At one point it felt like I was being convinced to lay down in the bed, to just let go and relax, that this idea of trusting the community and surviving in a grey area and not picking a side, not picking good or evil, was so stupid. I had to pick a side. I was being stubborn and stupid. I should just give in and give up and hurry up and fucking die.

But then part of me kept thinking, *Yes, it would be nice to give up, but you have to tell people about your story, about that creepy club in Vancouver, you can't just give up, this is bigger than just you.* These waves, these power struggles in my mind, they were so strong, I was so confused.

A doctor came in. At first, I wasn't sure if I could trust her, but she didn't have evil eyes and then I recognized her, I knew her, she had delivered Veronica. I had to trust her.

I was sobbing, holding my head, saying, "I am so confused, I don't know what to do." The brain fog was so strong.

The doctor wanted me to take some pills. She said they would calm me down and an ambulance would take me to Cranbrook for an assessment. The irony was not lost on me: Yesterday I wanted to be rushed to Cranbrook to see if I had some crazy brain tumour, and now that I was pretty sure I might only have one more day on earth, I really didn't want to spend my last day waiting around at the Cranbrook hospital. And I knew there would be a lot of waiting.

I chose to give in to the system. I took the pills and laid down on the hospital bed that was no longer my death bed. I kind of dozed off in a medication-induced calmness, and eventually got put onto a stretcher and hauled into an ambulance. I knew the ambulance driver and kind of knew the paramedic. The only thing I cared about was keeping my laptop safe. I trusted them. I also didn't have a choice.

They kept apologizing for the bumpy road on the way to Cranbrook, but I didn't really notice. I struggled to stay awake, to look out the little back window in the ambulance door, to remind myself what was happening. *You are on the way to the Cranbrook hospital, you can trust these people.* I still had my laptop. My kids were safe. That was all that really mattered.

AFTERNOON, MONDAY, SEPTEMBER 25TH, CRANBROOK HOSPITAL EMERGENCY ROOM

I arrived at the Cranbrook hospital around 1 p.m. The drugs were wearing off a bit.

Because I was a crazy person who was medicated, I think everyone talked freely and openly around me. The admissions nurse was pissed off that we were there, it was annoying to her to have to deal with another new patient. The Invermere hospital had phoned down, this wasn't a surprise, but she was still pissy about it. Because she was annoyed, she made up an excuse of having to do other things instead of filling in the admission paperwork, and she stormed off and left the paramedics standing there. They said, "This happens all the time." So, we all waited for more than half an hour before the pissy princess came back and angrily filled in the admission form.

An ER doctor mentioned something to everyone within ear shot: "They are doing another renovation and will move around some more walls, and we are going to lose another bed. Do you know that Invermere has more beds than we do?"

Wow, that didn't sound right.

Because they had no official beds left, they had a stretcher on wheels rolled over to a hallway area. They took me over for a CT scan, there was a lot of fussing around with key cards, I was still kind of groggy. After the CT scan was finished and I was back in the hallway area, a security guard arrived. I finally figured it out: The fussing with key cards and the doors, the security guard—that was because of me. I was in a secure section. Unbelievable.

My mom arrived. I was very lucky that she could and would drop work and everything to be my advocate. She was annoyed that the Invermere hospital didn't tell her when I was leaving. She wanted to be in Cranbrook when I arrived, but she drove fast and the ambulance drove slow, and I think she made pretty good time and really didn't miss much.

My limited experience over the last two days with the health care system was that no one has time to listen—well, maybe the security guard they brought in, he had literally nothing else to do. But the thing is, I'm not sure if he had any training on listening or counselling, and if you are afraid of police officers and authority, you don't want to start talking to someone in a uniform. The security guard assigned to my detail looked pretty harmless. If he was part of any big conspiracy, he was very low level. I probably could have talked to him, but he didn't look interested at all.

So we waited, we waited for hours. I knew we would be waiting there for a long time, I knew no one would tell us what was happening. I expected the lack of communication and the lack of personal care. At one point, I asked the security guard and a nurse if he could follow my mom and me to the nearby coffee shop in the lobby of the Cranbrook hospital so that I could buy a coffee and some food—you know, a supervised outing if you will. The answer was "no," that wasn't allowed.

I had not slept or eaten much for the last few days. I could have ended up in the psych ward just because I was "hangry." A very sweet lady, who is a Jehovah's Witness and a realtor, managed to get a care package with some granola bars, some fruit, and some water transported with me in the ambulance. She had gone through some health issues with her husband and was aware that they often didn't feed you or let you get food. This was such a blessing, and it made a huge difference in me not being hangry.

I wanted to make fun of the situation, how ridiculous it was. It got me pretty excited and worked up. My mom had to remind me a few times to calm down. While I was waiting, I sent emails to several UBCM senior staff who I knew personally. I explained that I was suffering from a mental health breakdown, and then I said I had some important ideas on how to transform UBCM and I wanted to meet with the executive in November. If I was going to be on Earth for longer than 24 hours or 7 days, then I had to play a role in doing some good, and UBCM was an excellent place to start.

After waiting for what I believe to be about 5 hours, it was after 6 p.m., a busy guy arrived. I never really got his name or credentials, but for lack of a better term, he was the shrink—and, I knew, he was my judge, jury, and executioner. His professional opinion of my condition was the sole determining factor of whether I was getting out of the hospital or getting locked up and drugged up in the psych ward.

He asked why I was in the hospital. I started talking about Vancouver and the creepy club. He cut me off. "I don't have time for this."

He had obviously listened to a lot of crazy manic stories before, and he knew this wasn't going to be a quick one. I tried to rationalize and negotiate with him and seek consent. I asked, "How long do you have?"

He said, "I don't know, I am on call."

"Well, since I am clearly not going anywhere, how about I start telling the story, and then if you have to go, you go, and then come back, and I will finish it."

He said, "No, it doesn't work that way."

He had a checklist he wanted to fill out. Another fucking checklist. It seemed like no one cared, they just wanted to fill out their stupid forms. I was frustrated. How could I truthfully answer his questions if he didn't have time to listen to the answers? The situation filled me with anger, but I knew I had to push it away. I took a deep breath. I had to do the best I could to tell him what he needed for his form.

I asked if I had a brain tumour and he said, "No, everything looks fine."

I tried to answer his questions in the shortest, most efficient way possible, in the calmest way possible. Enough truth, not all the truth. He wasn't friendly, he actually seemed like a jerk, but he seemed to know what he was doing. Objectively, he dealt with a lot of mentally ill people daily.

He suggested that this was likely a work-related burnout and prescribed a low-dose quick-release mood stabilizer that would act as a sleep aid. He informed us that all of the pharmacies in Cranbrook were already closed for the day, "so you can get the prescription filled tomorrow."

It was frustrating that I was such a risk to society that I had to be arrested under the Mental Health Act, transported by ambulance, guarded all day by a security guard, was not allowed to get food, but now, magically, I was no longer a risk and my condition was so unimportant that I couldn't get medication until the next day.

As my mom and I prepared to leave the hospital, I realized I had no shoes. Everyone was so busy deciding what I needed for medical care, so busy with checklists, they had forgotten to make sure my shoes were in the ambulance. I knew this was a simple mistake, there was a lot going on, but it was definitely an example of how the system operates. It seemed symbolic to me. A year earlier, when my dad was transported to Kelowna for an emergency pacemaker installation, they cut all of his shoelaces. I guess a bit faster than undoing the shoes—or was it? A complicated and busy system can forget the little human things, the things you need on the other side when you are recovering. Like your shoes.

My mom and I went for dinner at the Firehall in downtown Cranbrook. Jessie and Fred and all of the team are amazing at pulling off some cool concepts. It felt amazing to be free, to sip on some beer. I was a bit shaky, but I felt good. I felt free. It was actually kind of fun to walk around in my socks. I had a couple of hoppy beers and some nice food, and a really nice dinner with my mother. It was beautiful, something that I would never normally have made time for. It had been literally years, maybe since high school, since the two of us had a nice meal together in Cranbrook.

In the parking lot, as we were about to leave, there was a camper van and a young couple. The girl gestured for me to come towards them, to go into the van, in a seductive kind of way. I wasn't sure if

The Safe Word is PINEAPPLE!

that was real, it seemed kind of creepy, like another test. I ignored it and quickly got into the passenger seat of my mom's car.

During the drive back to Invermere, in the passenger seat with my mom's little dog Jasper on my lap, I typed up a Facebook message. I was operating on several levels: I wanted to explain some of my behaviour, I also believed that I needed to spread my message, to walk this fine line between sane and insane, and I needed as many "witnesses" in my community and in my social networks to vouch for me for what I felt could be upcoming judgements and to fight against future persecutions.

I believed that making myself a bit of a conspiracy theorist, spreading information far and wide in random ways, would be the best way to keep myself and my family safe. And if something sinister or mysterious were to happen to me, people would ask questions and look for answers. I decided that being public on Facebook was an important part of me telling my truth, it was a good way to get information out more efficiently, and I also thought it would be very useful to keep track of dates and thoughts for writing a future book.

It was also a test, a test of how free I was to express my opinions and to not be locked up. I should be free to post. If I somehow got censored, that would be proof that something wasn't right.

Posted to Facebook, 11:28 p.m. on Monday, September 25th:

> *Friends, family, neighbours, even to those that hate me: I have tried really really hard, I care so much, but one person can only do or carry so much. I recently suffered a mental health crisis, it was so scary, and I am not the same, I am trying to put the pieces together, but I need your help. If I am acting a little weird, please give me a bit of space to be weird, if my attention span is suffering, ask if I heard you. If you feel like it, give me a hug, if not don't, it doesn't matter. My kids are safe and*

> *I am safe. I am not going to hurt anyone, I know that. And I trust my community knows that. It might sound crazy, because it is, but if someone says I did something, ask me first or someone else if it was true. My only ask back from this community, if I am not harming anyone, there should never be a reason to lock me up. I believe in our systems and society norms, but declare I fiercely a freeman. Please keep it that way. I am actively looking to expand my friends, social, and support network. It's all I know right now. Thank you for those who can help and no judgement to those who can't.*

I knew my behaviour of running down the street with my daughter was not rational, but it also really bothered me that I was arrested under the Mental Health Act and that I was SO close to being institutionalized. I was so close to being held for days in a secure medical facility in another community, against my will.

As we were driving back to Invermere, I asked my mom, "Do you think my wife is really a demon? Was it a temporary spirit that took over her? Or could she part of some kind of conspiracy? Or was it all in my head?" Despite my mom believing deeply in various conspiracy theories, she assured me that my wife might be angry but was not a demon or a spy or some kind of secret agent. That was a relief!

But I still had some mistrust. I was going to stay at my mom's house for the foreseeable future.

CHAPTER 5

Un-Cult, Real Estate Breakup, and Pave the Damn Roads!

EARLY HOURS OF TUESDAY, SEPTEMBER 26TH, UN-CULT BC!

I was tired and unmedicated, but I was alive and I was free. I would only sleep for about an hour at a time, and it would feel like I had slept 8 hours. I fell back to sleep a few times before waking up around 2 a.m.

My mind was racing. Since I was still alive and had survived the first 24 hours, I might have a week (or maybe even 41 more years) left. It was time to start implementing my newfound knowledge and use my new powers to try to stop some kind of ultimate war, set to start around October 31st.

It occurred to me that the idea of a decentralized organization that operates a bit like a cult, but follows all laws, is a fairly good way for an outsider and non-believer to describe Jehovah's Witnesses. To me, the model of that organization is very effective at transmitting information and building small local communities and social circles. This type of organization is very independent and insular and would be very effective at resisting in the case of some kind of total war, or even a local war.

I was seeing a lot of patterns and messages in my life. It occurred to me that for much of my life I have been relatively close to current and former Jehovah's Witnesses. In my childhood, the lady who ran the daycare I attended was a devout Jehovah's Witness. I often grilled her on questions about the church, and a few times, on the rare Saturdays where we needed babysitting, my sister and I were brought to meetings and left in the back corner.

In my mid-twenties, I briefly dated and quickly fell in love with a beautiful, smart, and aloof young woman who had been raised in the Jehovah's Witnesses faith. She had agreed to get baptized when she was twelve, in return for getting permission to have her ears pierced. As an adult, she didn't believe in the teachings anymore, and while we were dating, she was "disfellowshipped" by the church—her family and everyone in the organization cut off all communication with her, effectively shunned her. Her mom initiated the disfellowship process. To me, it seemed incredibly cruel. My best friend Justin had a similar story with his family, as did the wonderful neighbour who protected Veronica.

To me, all these people are amazing. They have strong personal boundaries, strong morals, and are amazing friends, community members, and citizens. And they have had to overcome some very difficult and traumatic treatment from their families and from the "community" they were raised in. They have come out strong, well-rounded people, but I am not sure that all people are this strong.

In my mind, Jehovah's Witnesses would be the most efficient vehicle to spread my newly learned source code and life beliefs; however, the organization is very literal, dogmatic, and in my assessment, they got the order wrong. I believed they were forcing or encouraging people to choose community before family.

Around 3 a.m., I started crafting what could potentially become my new not-for-profit underground organization. My general concept was that this would be a bit of pledge to allegiance, an agreement to focus on shared values, not on difference of opinions. A sign that you weren't part of any polarizing conspiracy. I typed into the memo function of my Samsung cell phone while lying on my mother's couch. The couch is from the early 1990s, black fabric with a bit of an abstract, bright, colour print pattern—really not comfortable for sleeping on.

My concept was to take my new personal code of conduct, and my beliefs around the need to push against polarization, and try to spread them organically. I pictured that this could be on the membership card that people would carry in their wallets. I wanted it to be neutral enough that people with existing beliefs, existing allegiances to other religions and organizations, could still adopt these concepts.

Un-Cult BC

- Caring people (compassion first)
- REAL people (as honest as possible)
- REAL language (short, blunt, effective)
- WEIRD (funny, random, good weird)
- Organizational truth (decentralized, transparent, fair)

We are the common sense.

Radically boring & always law abiding.

Everything starts with informed consent, consent is always the first step.

We are the sweary and the smelly (but not too smelly.)

We want to help you to have more fun (but there are limits on the fun.)

We intend not to ever harm people or institutions, but we might offend some people, hopefully a lot of people will be deeply hurt and triggered by our messages. Good. That's on them.

We do not believe in complaint departments. When possible, complaints should be dealt with face-to-face by small groups directly involved.

RULES

- Building-block order: home, community,
- region & beyond
- Communication (thoughtful, compassionate, but also snappy & funny)
- Barter & trade, but not exclusively

I consent to be an Un-Cult member

I had many Facebook messages from friends and acquaintances offering encouragement and support after my public post about my mental struggles. One of the messages in my inbox was from Arjun Singh, a former Kamloops town councillor. I got to know Arjun through the time we spent working together on the UBCM executive board. I figured Arjun was the perfect partner to help with Un-Cult BC. He has strong personal values and beliefs in community, he doesn't take strong public partisan positions, and my impression is that he can see multiples sides and perspectives on issues and generally sees the good in people. He tries to collaborate, not divide.

I thought, *I need to float this Un-Cult BC idea to Arjun and see what he thinks.* So, at 4:18 a.m., I sent him my thoughts, describing it as "little networks of awesomeness."

Arjun later wisely responded that, to him, local government friends and colleagues are little networks of awesomeness, and he is not wrong about that. But I'm not sure if he shared my enthusiasm in the Un-Cult concept.

I floated the Un-Cult idea to a few people. No one specifically opposed it, but my tone and volume weren't perfect, I was pretty manic, and my very recent history of believing that I'd almost died, running down the street with my daughter and claiming my wife was a demon—it didn't exactly instil confidence in the messenger.

MORNING, TUESDAY, SEPTEMBER 26TH, THE REAL ESTATE BREAKUP

I felt kind of shaky, still not able to concentrate. I was very emotional, I felt that I had strong intuition, I believed that patterns were appearing everywhere, everything seemed kind of symbolic.

I didn't feel overly paranoid. I knew there were some things that I needed to accomplish, things that I needed to do. There were real life logistical considerations, a lot of money was at stake with real estate commissions and personally owned property that I was selling, and I had some significant bills and obligations to local trades for the renovation on the old Lordco (aka O'Lord) building in downtown Invermere.

I tried to get an appointment with my family doctor. The receptionist at the clinic knew me and seemed sympathetic and gave me a phone number for my doctor's private nurse, suggesting that I call her to try to get to see my doctor sooner. It made sense, but it was hard to navigate, it took a lot of concentration, and I had other appointments. I think I tried phoning later that afternoon—I'm not sure if I even left a message—I wanted to just walk in and get an appointment.

Around 10:30 a.m., my wife texted me and asked, *How are you doing?*

I responded with: *Weird, I am doing weird. How about you?*

I missed my wife and the kids, and I knew that I wasn't well enough to be fully welcome at home or around my kids yet, which hurt a lot.

The owner of my real estate office had asked about having a conversation the day before. I was completely ignoring any work emails and work-related text messages. I had no concentration, and staying alive and improving the world seemed far more significant. I knew that I couldn't function as a realtor at the time. I set up a face-to-face meeting for 11:30 a.m. that morning with the owner of my office and my managing broker.

I had a bad habit of being late for everything, but this day, I needed to have lots of time and it was very important for me to start the meeting on time. I arrived at the real estate office before 11 a.m., mustering all the concentration that I could, and I quickly put some numbers into a spreadsheet and did a quick estimate of cashflow coming in through commissions and property sales. My quick math, which definitely wasn't perfect, came to an amazing symbolic number. I had approximately $1,082,000 due to be coming in over the month of October. I was born in 1982; it was a sign (however, there were a lot of debts, bills, a building purchase, and taxes that needed to be covered by this incoming cash.)

I quickly typed up a word document:

Gerry & Rockies West Breakup

This might be for a little while, or this might be forever, I don't know. But unfortunately, I need a lot of distance right now, a lot. I love everyone on the team, and if I need anything from anyone, I will reach out.

I need time and space to figure out my shit. Whatever this shit is.

I so, so very much respect the ability to have this peaceful and mutually respectful departure or break.

I am so, so glad this not a hard breakup. I mean, it is hard, but not that hard. It could be harder.

What I would like:

- *I would like to be paid for fully closed deals but I need help to navigate those closures, I am willing to pay for that*
- *I would like to be paid a portion of the current pending deals, but only if that is fair, it doesn't have to be much*
- *I would like to copy anything/everything I want from the Google drive, I am willing to pay for that if you don't think that is fair*
- *I want to be fair and I want you to be fair*
- *Ideally, I get a couple of weeks to slowly move out of the office*

At the beginning of the meeting, I handed the paper to the owner of my office and my managing broker. I gave them a few minutes to read it, and then we started talking. The meeting was emotional, I was emotional. The owner of the office opened up about mental health issues in his own family. He suggested that this didn't need to be the end of a working relationship and that I didn't need to give up on real estate. We could take things easy for a bit and see how things worked out. This made a lot of sense, and I felt really good about the meeting. It seemed like we were on the same page and that we would be able to work out things in a fair way.

Because of the amount of work that the owner of the office and other people would have to do to help finish off some deals and find missing paperwork, I volunteered that for the month of October, instead of having a flat fee model for commission splits, I could go back to a percentage-split model that would result in the brokerage making more money. I felt this was only fair.

I knew that I was leaving a big, unorganized mess, and it would take work and effort to sort through everything. I had a lot of guilt for leaving things unfinished and not being able to "clean up my own mess." I wanted to try to help navigate it all, but I wasn't sure when I could help or how much I could help.

I talked about the desire to have time to drive a skid steer and move around dirt in my rural subdivision I was working on. And all of three of us agreed that for men, sometimes using equipment or plowing snow or doing certain tasks can be a form of meditation—mindless activities that can be useful in clearing the mind, thinking, and being alone.

It didn't come up at the meeting, and I was unaware of it until much later, but the day before, while I was probably travelling by ambulance to Cranbrook, my managing broker had blocked me from my work email. And I think around the same time I was kicked out from the office WhatsApp group. I wish that had been discussed at the face-to-face meeting; it surprises me that, during such an open and honest, heartfelt discussion, it wasn't mentioned. If I had known early on, if I had felt like I was part of the decision, it would have avoided a lot of future mistrust and paranoia. Also, had I remained part of the WhatsApp group, I would have felt more included and still welcome on the team.

Although I couldn't function in real estate, I had to try to manage and finish aspects of the commercial building renovation and my rural subdivision, and I was running everything through my one work email—a big mistake. Having the email blocked and not having access to older messages turned out to also be extremely annoying, and it made me dependent on my managing broker to forward over the emails he felt I needed to see.

AFTERNOON/EVENING, TUESDAY, SEPTEMBER 26TH

I went to the local Pharmasave and filled the prescription written by the shrink in Cranbrook. I took some of the medication right away. It was prescribed mostly as a sleep aid and was a quick-release medicine, but I was a bit confused on the dosage and timing. Instead of taking one or two pills before bed, I thought the proper dosage was a few pills throughout the day.

Standing at the Pharmasave, I was shocked to see a total of eight people behind the counter. And they were busy. The steady flow of people picking up medication really surprised me. They were literally pumping out the pills. It was eye-opening for me, as someone who had not been on any medication and who had this belief that Invermere and the surrounding area was a pretty healthy place. It was a stark realization that many people, whether for different physical, mental, or emotional conditions, are very dependent on a steady flow of medication.

That afternoon I attended a District of Invermere council (DOI) meeting. I disclosed to everyone that I was on medication and talked a bit about my experience through the weekend and about Cranbrook hospital the day before. I think it was emotional for everyone.

A number of Invermere council members and senior staff got COVID or were very sick after the UBCM Convention. Despite spending a lot of time with them, I was only sick in the head. Two of the council members and one of the staff members were attending the meeting virtually. Councillor Becker had her newborn baby on the screen, he was very cute. Little Harrison seemed to help a bit with making things not too heavy.

I had very little filter. I still didn't know how long I had to live. We had a frustrating situation through the winter and spring of 2023 with a major road in Invermere (13th Ave) not being paved, and some challenges with the general contractor on the project. DOI staff informed council at this meeting that the planned paving in other parts of town that we thought would happen in 2023 would probably not happen until 2024. There is a balance and a need for elected officials in strategic positions to not get too involved in operational details, and trust professional and paid consultants to do their jobs. But there can be times when it is necessary to ask tough questions, to break from polite decorum.

The lead engineer that Invermere contracts with was part of the meeting. I mentioned that we couldn't take back the mistakes and issues with the general contractor on the 13th Avenue project, but we needed to learn from those mistakes and make sure they weren't made again. I said that we needed to find a way to work with local contractors when possible because I didn't think they would have left the road in such a bad condition through the winter. And I expressed that it was unacceptable that the paving we had planned for 2023 wasn't going to happen on time, that we should be exploring competitor paving companies and all options to get the paving done.

Other council members echoed these thoughts and added their own perspectives. We had a very honest and sincere meeting. Everyone was respectful; it felt like we were talking in very real terms and we weren't allowing excuses and justifications to be the answers to problems. We started the meeting on time and ended the meeting on time. It was one of the best council meetings I have ever been part of. We were a team, we were being effective, and we were holding staff, consultants, and contractors accountable. The paving, and even some additional portions, ended up getting done in the fall of 2023.

After the council meeting, I picked up some grocery-store Chinese food and went to my mom's house. I knew that I had a few nice hoppy IPA beers stashed in her fridge. Upon arriving at my mom's house, the lights were on, the music was going, there was a big pot of homemade chicken soup simmering on the stove; but neither my mom nor her little dog Jasper were there.

I cracked opened the Fernie Brewing Co.'s Thunder Meadows IPA beer, went to heat up the food, and then started laughing to myself, remembering that my mom didn't have a stupid microwave. I turned on the oven and looked for a casserole dish. We were going to have to go old school.

My mom had a radio show playing, *Lionel's Vinyls* from independent Alberta radio station CKUA. Lionel was playing classic rock, and the music was good. I cranked it up. I tasted the soup simmering on the stove. It was really good. Some of the vegetables were still a little crunchy, but it was edible. I sipped my beer, and I smiled.

I was basically having a little party in my mom's house. The exact same house that I'd lived in from the age of 10 until graduating high school (and then again for summers during and right after college). I felt like a teenager. The music, the location—it brought me back in time. I had access to all these old memories. A lot of the people who had reached out to me on Facebook were old friends, people I hadn't talked to since basically high school, which was bringing back so many more old memories.

This moment at my mom's house really felt like part of a rebirth—maybe I was at a juvenile/teen stage. But it was fun. It was beautiful.

I ate my grocery-store Chinese food, crunched on the soup vegetables, and enjoyed a really good meal by myself with classic rock blaring in the background. It was about then that my mom and Jasper returned home from their walk. I turned down the music. She was happy to see me, happy to see me happy (and not doing anything too crazy).

I posted a picture of the pill bottle and asked the world of Facebook friends if taking this medication was a good idea or not. It seemed like a good way to be transparent, prove that I was on medication, but also to stimulate some discussion. This was the first post where I started to understand that a lot of people know what works well for them (or what they have always done). People will very strongly project, encourage, or dump onto you their solutions or their ideas. I got some advice, some people recommended other types of medication, some people said it was fine, some people recommended herbal alternatives. I got a mixed bag of strongly held opinions.

CHAPTER 6
Paranoia and Persecution

WEDNESDAY, SEPTEMBER 27TH

After 8 hours of deep sleep, I woke up (in reality, it had only been an hour). I tried to post about my thoughts on trans rights and dicks versus clicks, but it wasn't well written, I couldn't fully articulate my thoughts. After waking up again, around 5 a.m., I realized that I was seeing so many parallels to George Orwell's classic dystopian novel. It was so symbolic that his book was titled *1982*, the same year that I was born. I posted on some buy and sell groups that I wanted to buy copies of the book. Several people corrected me: It was actually called *1984*. Other people didn't seem to notice. It seemed like a funny test to leave my reference to it as 1982.

I stopped into the clinic in person, and I was ushered into a room and was able to see my family doctor almost immediately, with no appointment. It wasn't until later that I realized how lucky and privileged that was (and that I even have a family doctor). He reviewed the prescription from the Cranbrook shrink and indicated that he didn't love quetiapine, but since I was already on it, he would continue this with a second higher-dose, low-release prescription. He also prescribed Apo Valproic.

I went to fill the prescription at the Pharmasave, and the pharmacist and co-owner Keith was very patient with me. He told me he had to wait until the clinic faxed the prescription over. In 2023, it seems very surprising to me that prescriptions rely on a fax machine. I talked with Keith about the volume of people I saw the other day, and he commented that the volume of medication they are sending out the door has increased dramatically since COVID. I asked Keith if he would be comfortable with me videotaping him and if he wanted to do a documentary on mental health. He seemed interested.

He invited me into a little office and told me that a lot of people took similar medication to the prescriptions I was filling. At the time, that made me feel good, less strange or weird. But it was also concerning. Why did everyone need to be medicated? Why had it increased so much?

My wife invited me to come over to our house. She was happy that I was seeing my doctor and getting medication. After talking for a bit, she agreed to let me try staying at the house. I spent most of the day in my bed, sleeping a bit and responding to messages on Facebook and posting things online.

It felt like my energy level was somewhat connected to the sun. When the sun was shining, I felt so energetic, and then when it got cloudy or the sun wasn't out, I felt drained and a bit anxious, like I had to recharge. Sometimes I rested for 20 minutes, sometimes I would fall into a deep sleep for an hour. When I woke from a nap, I would feel very well rested but totally disoriented to what time it was. I noticed that there were waves of paranoia, periods where it really felt like someone or something was out to get me, almost like waves of energy attacking me, and then those periods would pass.

keep pushing baxk enough?
= let your imagination go a little wild, but not too wild
÷ look for some patterns but not too hard?

That afternoon I posted a similar style of writing all over social media, with purposely misspelled words. It was fun, a joke code, and I thought I was poking and teasing the AI machines and their masters. To the outside, it probably looked like I had really cracked.

The owner of my real estate office phoned me and told me that they needed to suspend my licence. If I remember correctly, it was very much mentioned as a pause or a break, and it was suggested that this was being done to protect me.

At the time, and in the moment, I was in a positive "love and compassion" mood and looking for signs and patterns. I think that initially I said something like: "I need boundaries"— basically some guidance on how far to push my desire to advocate for change and call bullshit on systems. I knew that my tone and volume were not perfect, some of my points were not landing, people were not picking up what I was trying to put down, so I was open to input and guidance from people. I needed people to tell me when I was going too far or acting too weird.

But my mood changed when I received an email from my managing broker, which I only skimmed. It hurt too much to read the full thing (and it was still really hard to concentrate on emails and longer blocks of text).

Gerry,

First off, I want to again stress how much my heart goes out to you at this time. I do understand that you need this time to sort things for yourself and it pains me to have to finalize things in this way. I do however feel this is the best for your protection and ours. I have notified

BCFSA and AIR that we have surrendered your license for now.

I do have to ask that you must remove all references to the brokerage and real estate from all websites, social media, vehicles, billboards and advertising of any kind as soon as possible. Also please refrain from any conduct that could be considered realtor -related with anybody. FYI I will arrange to have the billboard removed from my property. Let me know if I can help with any of the other things.

I cannot stress enough how much I care for your well being right now. I hope you can find your way to happiness or at least contentment whatever that means to you.

Do not hesitate to reach out to me if you need my help.

Your friend,

I checked my phone. I was no longer part of the office WhatsApp group chat. I checked my work email. I couldn't log in. It hurt so much.

My identity, almost every waking minute of the last 5, almost 6 years, was being a realtor. It had taken awhile to build, but I had become the top agent in my office and one of the top agents in the Royal LePage franchise system (for individual agents not part of a team). I never thought I would suddenly not be licensed, not be successful. I never thought I would be asked to pull down all of my branding, to go dark. I never thought I would be eliminated from the team.

In BC, there is a rule that says that if you are not licensed, all of your branding is supposed to come down immediately. I believe the intent behind this rule is if you have a licence suspension for doing something wrong (in these situations, the start date for suspension is negotiated and known long in advance), or if

The Safe Word is PINEAPPLE!

you choose to quit or retire, your branding should come down. I don't think the rules ever considered a serious medical situation, whether that be mental or physical.

My managing broker hinted that there were agents from another office threatening to file a complaint against me and/or the brokerage. I responded with a request for time. There was no way that I could navigate getting signage down, have logos scraped off my truck. I had already asked my friends and family to do so much for me. There was no way that I could put this onto them. And it didn't feel right. I wanted to fight this rule, not comply with it. I wasn't trying to sell any real estate, I knew I couldn't function as a realtor at that moment, and I wasn't trying to be one. But I didn't want to be silenced, I didn't want to be hidden as a person, and I didn't want to be cancelled.

I wanted to be an advocate for mental health. I wanted to prove that I had no shame or guilt. I wanted to fight against bullshit and broken systems. I still had no idea how long I would be living, or whether I would get locked up. Taking down signs seemed like a waste of time and submitting to a stupid rule. If I had died, or was in a serious car accident, or suddenly had an aggressive cancer, would there have been a mad rush to take down signs? Would there be other agents threatening to file complaints? Probably not.

I wanted social connection and normalcy so badly. Even if I couldn't function in real estate, I wanted to be able to go to the office and try to start piecing back together my life. But now it didn't feel like I was welcome at my office, I wasn't part of the team. At the face-to-face meeting we had the day before, it had felt like we were on good terms. The owner of the office had suggested that this didn't need to be a full breakup with real estate. The actions were different than the words.

Over the next week or more, having my work email blocked and having them terminate me fed into paranoia loops. Were they going to rip me off for commissions owing? Was this part of some bigger persecution or effort to silence or hurt me? Was there some bigger conspiracy against me?

Earlier that year, I had bought a big old cube van, got my name and logo plastered on it. Originally the concept was a big rolling billboard, a free van for community groups and people to use when moving. But throughout the year, the usage and the demand for the van had been amazing. It was important to me to keep my website live, to keep the booking of the van going. Over the next few days, I did a quick edit to my website and took down references to real estate and kept it live as a booking platform for the community van.

The experience with my brokerage was such a contrast compared to the experience with the DOI. Although I later decided it would be a good idea to take a short leave from council (I think I only missed one committee and one council meeting), I always felt welcome, my email was never blocked, I always felt like I was part of the team.

I know that other elected officials have had much tenser council relationships and have not had the same level of respect and support from fellow council members or from their municipal administration. I am very grateful for the relationships, support, and general lack of freaking out from the DOI team. I wish this experience to all elected officials; the role can be challenging enough. I can't imagine how terrible it would have been for me if the DOI team had reacted in a similar way to my real estate office.

I wonder if that council meeting on the Tuesday, about being vulnerable and explaining my story face-to-face, made a difference to how people perceived me? If I had had the same in-person interactions with all the agents in my office, would that have made a difference? Most of them hadn't seen me in person and were only seeing what I was posting online, or what people were saying behind my back. Or, with it being commission sales and a competitive environment, was I naïve? Maybe there really never was much of a team, maybe there were a lot more people cheering for my downfall, waiting to pick up the pieces and the business?

Upon reflection and with benefit of a clear mind and time, I know the intentions of the people at my former office were pure. They weren't trying to harm me; they were trying their hardest to protect the organization and manage risk. Everyone was in shock. Everything had happened so quickly. And I have to accept my share of responsibility. I was not perfect. I took on more work than I could effectively handle. I wasn't always easy to work with, and I wasn't always a team player.

I hope that real estate brokerages and regional real estate boards can look out for the warning signs of agent mental health and burn out, and ideally put in policies and mechanisms that can allow someone to take a break without having to completely cancel them and end their career. Unfortunately, it seems like some policies on social media and morality are going the other direction, making it easier to cancel anyone who may act erratically. We need to leave room for people to be human, to be honest/transparent, and to make mistakes. I hope that there are very few agents who would be eager to file a complaint and kick someone when they are down.

EARLY EVENING, WEDNESDAY, SEPTEMBER 27TH

I got to see my kids for the first time since Monday morning. It took a few minutes for them to be comfortable. I read a story to Veronica, and I cuddled with both of them on the couch. It felt so good to be with them.

We tried to settle into normal routines. One unhealthy evening routine I had used in the last few years, when busy with real estate, was letting the kids pick YouTube kids shows on my laptop. While they were watching shows, I could rush downstairs to my desktop computer to finish a portion of the pile of work I hadn't finished yet, send the electronic signings for pressing offers, respond to some emails, make a phone call or two.

This evening, I stayed with the kids as they watched a Minecraft–themed show. The announcer guy was cocky, there were subtitles, and then there were secondary subtitles—words spelled wrong, like how I had been spelling them all day. The secondary subtitles kind of waved and faded a bit, looking different, looking manipulated.

The announcer guy continued: "This noob thinks he is so tough, but we can easily get into his house, he hasn't even set a trap, I bet the door is unlocked."

The flickering secondary sub-title: *Gud luk gitting out . . . if u evan kan.*

The whole show felt directed at me, like AI or whoever was controlling it was sending me a message. A threat!

I took pictures with my phone, my heart was pounding. This was not cool. I was seeing this in real time. Technology had been so glitchy, and at the worst possible time, things were not working and had been so hard to navigate. And now this. I was sure that someone was messing with this show. I slammed the laptop closed and told the kids they couldn't watch that show. Upset, they ran to their mom.

I posted on a community Facebook group asking for a night watch. I gave the slightly wrong address to my house, changing the last number. I tagged my sister's husband on the post. My sister texted me immediately saying not to tag him. My wife told me to take the post down. The address that I thought was fake was actually a neighbour's house (a bit of a distance away. We have an empty lot beside us, I never realized the numbering was so weird). I felt terrible. I was so anxious and upset, I thought I was being kind of sneaky changing one number of the house address, but here I was potentially harming other people accidentally. I deleted the post.

I had been turning my phone off and ignoring it for big periods of time. That night, I unplugged the internet modem and turned my phone off. We also decided, going forward, to read with the kids before bed instead of watching YouTube videos.

CHAPTER 7
Free Gerry's Shoes

THURSDAY, SEPTEMBER 28TH

I woke up with energy. I tried doing a Peloton workout for the first time, but it glitched on me. I was still having challenges with technology.

That morning, I wanted to feel comfortable and feel good, and I didn't care what I looked like. I put on my favourite pair of jeans and an untucked dress shirt, and broke all fashion rules by wearing socks and sandals. I still had not gotten my shoes back. The sun was coming out. It was going to be a beautiful day.

We walked in the field between our neighbourhood and Eileen Madson Primary School (the same school I attended as a child). As we got close to the school, my wife told me I wasn't allowed on the property. I wasn't sure if this rule came from her or from the school, or both, but either way, I couldn't fight against all the rules. I had to accept this one. It was more important to stay with my family and spend time with my kids. They were safe at school, and I had no reason to cause any fear or issues by being on the grounds, so I stopped at the gate by the play field and said goodbye to my kids.

I drove to the Invermere hospital. I was going to start the process of getting my shoes back. I wanted to document the process, how complicated it can be. I thought it could be symbolic of how complicated and bureaucratic many of our government systems have become.

I was feeling strong, ready to start changing the world! I changed my Facebook profile picture to a picture of poo in the toilet, I changed my description to "poo stirrer upper," and I made my Facebook profile public.

In front of the hospital, I filmed myself ranting, explaining how I made almost $1 million a year selling real estate in Invermere (that figure is a bit exaggerated and definitely not net income). I said I had blown up my career, explained that I was going to film the process of trying to get my shoes back, but I would ask for consent to film. I was passionate, I was emotional, I was manic.

At the check-in desk for the non-emergency side of the Invermere hospital, I recognized both people working there. I explained that my shoes had been forgotten at the hospital on Monday when I was taken to Cranbrook and that I would like to film the process of me asking for my shoes back and what that process looks like.

One of the women commented on why filming wasn't allowed: "Gerry, you know there are a lot of privacy rules because this is a . . . public . . . facility." In the middle of making the comment, she realized how ironic or contradictory what she was saying was. I smiled. It was part of my point.

They decided they had to call a manager. I took a seat. A manager arrived a few minutes later. She suggested that any request to film would have to be decided by someone above her.

"We both know if you run this up the Interior Health Authority hierarchy, the answer will be no," I explained firmly and calmly. "This should be a local decision, you should have the power to decide."

She did not seem to agree with me.

I realized that I was putting this poor lady on the spot and had not given any advance notice of this request. A surprise situation did not seem consistent with my belief in having consent. I said, "Surprising you with this isn't fair. I will come back tomorrow morning around this time and then you can decide how to handle this."

I had created a little bit of scene in the waiting room, but I wanted to have witnesses, I wanted people to notice the conversation. I was having a public conversation in a public facility. I wasn't being abusive, and I wasn't being aggressive.

I realized that the chair I had sat in was reserved for people that needed a "boost." I think it means someone who needs help getting up or down. It was another example of how self-centred and oblivious I can be. I thought it was funny that I never noticed the sign and sat in the wrong chair. I asked someone nearby to take a photo of me. I felt like I needed a boost. I needed to take more medication and go back to the safety of my home. I was feeling tired.

I posted a follow-up video about the lack of success on filming the return of my shoes. Justin saw the social media posts, and he asked about coming over to my house for lunch; he would bring some food. This felt like an intervention. I knew this would be a tough conversation, but he was coming, whether I was ready for him or not.

Justin is a strong, action-focused entrepreneur. You can trust him completely. He is very loyal, very logical, and very ADHD. Justin has three kids and years of experience being a boss, running restaurants and various businesses. In the past, Justin has had other friends crack mentally—drug-induced in those cases. Justin has no problem taking charge and managing a situation. And for many people, that's what they need: a boss and someone to take over and make decisions. Unfortunately, that is not me. I am fiercely independent, a bit of a lone wolf when it comes to finances and business decision-making.

Justin was challenging me. "Dude, you don't have any special powers, you aren't some kind of 'second coming,'" "I'm pretty sure no one is after you," "Who has control of your bank accounts and your finances?"

I pushed back on what I could, but some of what he was saying I couldn't argue with. And when Justin is determined or convinced that he is right, there is a fierce amount of power with those convictions. He can be very convincing, or at least impossible to argue with.

My memory of the conversation is blurry. I had noticed that the amount of medication I was taking was now starting to impact my short-term memory. Even my thought process seemed a bit delayed. I remember thinking: *Justin is trying to manage me.*

By time the conversation ended, the sun had gone behind some clouds, the weather had turned. I felt even more drained and completely depressed. Maybe this was all in my head and I had destroyed my real estate career for no reason? Was I just crazy? Was this all my fault?

AFTERNOON, THURSDAY, SEPTEMBER 28TH

After a short nap, I felt recharged. I knew that Justin cared and he wasn't trying to manage me, he was trying to bring me back down to earth. I needed to be able to listen to friends and family. I needed outside perspective. I didn't have to agree with everything that they said, but I needed to consider their perspectives. And I was fucking lucky to have them.

For a long time, I had secretly been jealous of hipsters with record players. Perhaps inspired by the classic rock music playing a few days earlier at my mom's house, I decided I wanted to try to buy a record player and some records. I think it was a bit of a push back against Justin asking who was controlling my finances—*Yeah, I am, and I'm going to waste some money on a fucking record player.*

My wife warned me there might not be any record players for sale in Invermere, but I headed downtown on an adventure. It felt amazing to walk around downtown Invermere and have face-to-face conversations. In a sense, it felt like the 1980s, like my childhood. Very analog, very real and safe. Being free to do this was definitely part of my recovery. It made me appreciate locals, people I knew, and that I was in my hometown. I went to a number of stores, including some second-hand ones, and bought a couple of LPs and had some great conversations. But it turns out that my wife was right: There were no actual record players available.

That evening, I got a text message from an ex-girlfriend. Not just any ex-girlfriend, but the one that I had never really gotten over. The one where it had been years of hoping to have her reach out, hoping to have a connection again. It was amazing, like this really was my best life and my perfect life, heaven on earth! I really had redesigned my life and without even knowing it, she was part of my life again! I felt god-like. It was very symbolic because she grew up as a Jehovah's Witness and she'd been screwed over by her family and the church. She would understand the points I was trying to make.

In reality, she was just being a good person and worried about me. Over the next week and a bit, she got a lot of text messages and some manic emails and attempts at writing. In addition to explaining my various ideas, including Un-Cult, and wanting to radically change the religion of Jehovah's Witnesses, I explained that I was working on improving my relationship with my wife, which meant me and her (the ex-girlfriend) would probably never end up together. I also explained that I always hedge my bets, so you never know for sure. Maybe one day we would? Looking back on it, I'm surprised she kept talking to me.

MORNING, FRIDAY, SEPTEMBER 29TH

I woke up and it was dark and a bit chilly. I grabbed some warm clothes without really looking or paying attention. The first shirt I grabbed was a fleece, plaid button-up shirt with the Royal LePage logo (a past Christmas gift from my former office) and the other was a comfortable hoodie with the UBCM logo on it (another gift during my time on the executive).

There had been no response from my emails to various UBCM staff. I knew the week after the convention was a time when staff might be off work recovering, or trying to catch up on things that transpired through the week. And when you open an email disclosing that you are having a mental health breakdown, that can leave people unsure of how to engage or respond, and my specific request to meet with the UBCM executive at their November meeting was not a normal request. Many valid reasons to receive no response, but it still hurt at the time to have not heard anything from anyone. (I later received a response, including a personal call from the UBCM president.)

I was disappointed and frustrated. Also, in a sense, I was mourning my lack of involvement and importance with both organizations. It seemed so symbolic that these were the two pieces of clothing that I grabbed for comfort and warmth. They are part of my identity and history (and objectively comfortable and warm clothing). I made a social media post with pictures of both, saying I was lightly shaming both organizations.

I tried to post about a rally. I wanted to do a joke satire rally in front of the Invermere hospital to demand my shoes back. I thought it would be fun and funny. The paranoid side of me was trying to test boundaries and see how safe I was. If I possessed some powerful information and was starting to host rallies, they—or whatever evil forces—wouldn't be very happy about this. I could get locked up, or worse—somehow eliminated.

I had a doctor appointment scheduled at 9:30 a.m. and Justin wanted to attend. He told me to delay my hospital rally until after the appointment. I was too smart for that. I was doing the rally between walking the kids to school and the doctor appointment, while he was too busy to stop me.

While walking with the kids and wife to school, I was emotional. I believed that there could be dozens, maybe more, who would show up to the rally, and that I could get arrested or, potentially and by a small chance, be assassinated. I was still unsure of my deal for more time on Earth and how much time I would get. This could be a suicide mission. My heart was pounding. I didn't want to die, but I had to test how free I was. If I was truly free, if there was no one after me, I should be able to do goofy little rallies without the fear of being arrested or harmed.

Wearing my plaid Royal LePage shirt, UBCM hoodie, and socks with sandals—this was my pride parade. This was me taking back my strength and autonomy in my own quirky and manic way. I was making a point about my shoes, I wasn't happy about these organizations, I wasn't happy about going crazy, I wasn't happy about how complicated many systems are. I was proving that I could speak my mind and be a pain in the ass, be a "poo stirrer upper" (a shit disturber), this shouldn't be shunned or silenced, and this definitely isn't illegal. I stood in front of the hospital. Alone. There was no crowd of people, there was no real reaction or traction on social media. I was just a crazy person posting crazy stuff. People were staying away.

I had decided that any outcome that didn't involve me getting arrested or killed was a success, even if no one showed up. One sweet lady who had messaged me earlier to ask a few questions showed up. I believe she has had her own struggles with mental health. I don't think she really understood what I was attempting to do, but she was there to support me. As we stood there, a former Invermere town councillor, friend, and past political activist, Bob Campsall, arrived at the hospital. He also had no idea what I was talking about, but he joined anyway.

The three of us walked into the Invermere hospital shortly after 9 a.m., and the ladies at the admissions desk were smiling. They were expecting me, and they were so proud to hand over a brown paper bag with my shoes and a computer charger, which I had forgotten about. Simply getting my shoes back was not what I was trying to accomplish, but it does prove the advantages of living in a small town, of knowing a lot of people, of being privileged. I doubt getting my shoes back from the Kelowna hospital would have been as easy or as successful. Although the rally was not understood, I was grateful for my two witnesses.

I was so focused on going to the doctor appointment that I actually forgot the brown bag with the shoes and charger outside the hospital, but my wife showed up at the hospital parking lot and with her help, we made it to my doctor appointment, and my shoes eventually made it home!

At the appointment, my family doctor recommended increasing the dosage of the medicine he had prescribed and he warned me that I was walking a fine line between being institutionalized and being able to stay at home. I don't remember this, but apparently he explained that I was in psychosis and that things should normalize after about a week or two.

AFTERNOON, FRIDAY, SEPTEMBER 29TH

That afternoon, my sister delivered a record player and a few records that her husband's dad had in storage. I had never actually played a record on my own before. My kids and I learned how to drop the needle at the same time. To share this experience, and to have a technology that is so simple that Veronica could operate it on her own, was a beautiful experience.

The classic rock music improved my mood. The songs seemed symbolic, and the lyrics made so much sense. They were pushing against authority. I felt like I was on the same level as some of these artists were in the 60s and 70s, and objectively, I was on a fair bit of medication and potentially coming off of some weird drug trip.

At several points, my life felt like a movie. When I played "The Sound of Silence" by Simon & Garfunkel, it felt like the soundtrack to the end of the movie—to me winning, to being alive, being free, being sane, to being recovered. Playing the song on vinyl while sipping a hoppy beer, it filled me with energy, it gave me motivation, and it gave me hope.

I had a vision of getting out on my little 18-foot pontoon boat that I had just bought weeks earlier. If I could be mentally and physically strong enough to bring the boat out, and free enough to be allowed to do it, if I could bob around on the water, then I would know I was winning, that the world, society, Invermere, and I weren't too far gone. That maybe things were normal, maybe I didn't have any special powers, and maybe no one was after me or my family.

CHAPTER 8

Meeting With the MLA and Faking It Until You Make It

SOCIAL MEDIA REACTIONS AND ENERGY ATTACKS

It felt so important to post publicly, to test my freedom of speech, but it came with a number of costs. Clearly some of my early posts had contributed to my former brokerage terminating and cancelling me, which had some big financial implications. But there was also an emotional cost to navigating the responses. There were some great connections, virtual conversations with people I had not talked to in years, conversations with ex-girlfriends, some really amazing human connections. But there were also some negative reactions, what I would describe as virtue signalling and people who were very easily triggered. Several messages went along the lines of: "Let me know if you need anything, but you really shouldn't use the word 'crazy' to describe yourself, that can be very offensive."

"FUCK YOU! I am fucking crazy!" I wanted to say this back in response, but I didn't. It seemed strange to me that describing myself as crazy would be triggering. The word has many meanings and degrees of seriousness. By scolding me on the use of this word, did they think they were helping me?

Because I was opening my mind to anything and everything, including conspiracy theories and evil in the world, I experienced an interesting shift: My enemies became my friends, those with deep conspiracy theory beliefs were very welcoming and accepting, very open to having me learn more about their beliefs. And some of the people who were aligned with my old beliefs were convinced that I had cracked and were the first to distance from me or try to silence me. People from all sides, however—friends, family, everyone—were telling me to stop posting on social media. The more people told me to stop, the less I wanted to. This was my independence; it was a test of how free I was. If I wasn't allowed to post, that would be a real sign that things were not right.

During the last week of September and first few weeks of October, it seemed like so many minor celebrities and semifamous people were dying—like, every day there was another person. They seemed like good people, not perfect people but good people. Many of the deaths were freak accidents. I had a theory that maybe grey people were being pushed to pick a side. Maybe they were being tricked into opting out of staying alive and staying on Earth. It made me question whether our subconscious is powerful enough that a person can choose to die. And if that is the case, could some evil force trick people into choosing that?

It felt like huge waves of energy were being directed at me. The waves of energy would then produce anxiety or paranoia. These waves would come often after waking up from a nap, or sometimes later in the evening.

I reached out to people who I knew were into mystical and supernatural beliefs. Similar to my conversation with my mom about conspiracy theories, I was looking for high-level concepts and explanations for what I was going through. I was open to new belief systems. Some of what I learned was useful, like blessing the medication to take away any harmful reactions, me firmly declaring to anyone/everyone/no one that my house was a safe place and they had no right to attack me—these seemed to have some positive effects. But when some of the people started to get really specific about spirit guides, reincarnation, and pushing me to do certain meditations—well, it just got too detailed and nuanced for me. I was happy to learn about the high level, and about the common values, but I didn't want to be pushed into a belief system or made to pick a side. And as soon as I felt like I was being pushed or pulled into a camp, I pulled back.

SATURDAY, MORNING, SEPTEMBER 30TH

Although my attempts to reach out to some staff at UBCM were not initially successful, Columbia River–Revelstoke MLA Doug Clovechok (who I lost the 2017 election to) and his wife, RDEK Area F Director Susan Clovechok, gracefully agreed to meet me for breakfast at Rocky River Grill, a restaurant owned by my friend Justin and where I had worked briefly after losing the election and while taking the real estate course.

I rambled on for nearly two hours, explaining my story about nearly dying and the visions that I saw. Doug and Susan were supportive and vulnerable. Doug talked a bit about some of his health struggles, and they recommended a counsellor in Cranbrook. At the end, I was emotionally and physically drained, I felt shaky and a bit paranoid. I no longer thought it would be a great idea to drive home. I called my wife for a ride.

Doug was going to pay for his breakfast. And then Susan was going to pay for my breakfast. From what Doug explained, the paperwork and process of expensing another meal wasn't worth it, and there was much scrutiny to expenses. It seemed so ridiculous to me that a MLA couldn't buy breakfast for a constituent, that the rules would get in the way of that kind of connection. Clearly, in the private sector, it wouldn't be a question and it wouldn't be difficult to expense. I don't think any corruption in our system is happening with a $15 breakfast. I paid for everyone's meal and said that Doug should point out how stupid the rules are. Expense forms not worth filling out wasn't the solution to corruption or inefficiencies. If we can't trust our elected officials or civil servants with small expenses, how can we trust them with big decisions?

When my wife and kids arrived, we left my truck at the restaurant and drove home. I was struggling with the increased level of medication. Time was hard to navigate, and I would often wake up in cold sweats and be very disoriented about what time it was. It felt like everything I was doing was potentially being monitored. One thing that was reassuring was that nothing I did or said was a secret; in fact, I wanted it to be shared far and wide.

But I was craving some analog, fewer digital options, and redundancy and backup. I asked my wife to buy an old-school wall clock that ran on batteries, and an analog wristwatch so that when I woke up at weird times, I could see what time it was without having to turn on my cell phone or some kind of digital device. I also asked her to buy an external hard drive so I could back up data, extra printer ink so that I could print hardcopies. I had enough supplies to last in case I was put under house arrest, which I thought could be a reality.

One could debate how functional of a family we were before. I was so busy working that I wasn't around much, and even when I was physically around, I wasn't necessarily mentally available and really paying attention to the kids. I wasn't sure now how to be a good parent before. But now, now that I wasn't 100% healthy, I really didn't know what to do. But I had access to all these memories from my childhood, and I started mimicking the way my parents parented me, the way that Glady treated the kids at daycare. I decided to "fake it until I made it" and pretend, in a sense, that I was reliving the 1980s.

That afternoon, we started playing Dog-Opoly, a dog-themed version of Monopoly. I loved Monopoly as a kid (my sister jokingly blames it for my obsession with real estate as an adult). It felt really cool to share this with my kids. I still wasn't sure how long I was going to be alive or normal, and if I could teach them a little bit about real estate and negotiating, that felt important. Also, teaching them to count money and do simple math seemed liked solid 1980s parenting. It took all my concentration to play the game. Counting change back and dealing with the money was a struggle, forcing my drugged-up brain to work. It pushed away some of the fog, but it was hard. I noticed my impaired cognitive abilities, how cloudy and slow my brain was.

That evening, during another paranoid wave, I tried resetting a lot of my passwords to email accounts; however, technology was still very difficult to navigate, and I almost locked myself out of some accounts. I wanted to post on some other social media platforms, like X/Twitter, but it was so glitchy, almost evil, and I removed it from my phone. My impression was that Apple and Google were very secure, but their security on resetting passwords was so tight and circular that it was difficult to navigate. Samsung and Telus seemed glitchy and weak.

I never thought I would, but I signed up for Truth Social. It was by far the easiest platform to navigate. It might've been designed for dumb people and therefore designed to be simple. Too bad that the rest of the world has to be so complicated and hard to navigate. It can leave some people behind. Although I could sign up for Truth Social, I never posted anything there. It was a backup emergency social media outlet, if for some reason I was blocked or banned or locked out of all the other ones.

It did give me pause to consider Donald Trump in another way. I had viewed him as a not-so-smart narcissistic asshole, but what if he really was some kind of freedom fighter draining the swamp and exposing some large-scale conspiracy? What if Truth Social really was a truly independent platform? It was interesting to legitimately consider a polar-opposite view to one that I'd held for a long time. It gave me some perspective on how some other people think. It is undeniable that certain famous people do have an immense amount of power and they seem to accomplish unbelievable things. The list of examples is endless, but I thought specifically about Donald Trump and Elon Musk. Maybe they did have some kind of divine, superhuman powers. Or maybe they'd made some kind of deal with some evil force, basically a deal with the devil.

EVENING, SATURDAY, SEPTEMBER 30TH

I received a text from a girl I know. I think that her siblings have had some challenges with drugs in the past, maybe the present. She had asked me a few weeks earlier to try to help her find a place to rent, and I had ignored her; there are very few rentals available. When I saw a text coming in from her, I felt guilty for ignoring her, but the text made me stop what I was doing because it seemed so creepy: *Can you pretty please bring my dress in the morning it's in grandma's closet.*

It was so cryptic and weird. Initially I felt scared. But then I felt angry. I thought, *She must know what I am going through, why would she send a message like that to me? That isn't funny—it's mean. She is trying to fuck with me, and that's bullshit.* I wanted to lash out, but I realized I wasn't in the right state of mind. I ignored it, I parked it, and I went to sleep.

I woke up around 11 p.m. and wrote back: *Amanda, that was a really weird message to send.*

She wrote back the next day: *Oh my god, that's the last time I ever use Siri, I was asking my daughter to get my dress for my sister's wedding, I am so sorry that got sent to you.*

I started writing and analyzing. Compared to earlier that afternoon, I felt very lucid, my mind felt clearer. Since there had been no response from UBCM staff, I emailed some of the current executive members. (I had a kind and thoughtful response back the next morning from Vancouver City Councillor Pete Fry, and later I had a response back from UBCM staff and a phone call with the UBCM president.)

I started to describe myself not as crazy, but as brain injured—something had happened to my brain. It was going to take time to recover. Maybe this was all triggered by drugs at that creepy club? And now I was taking lots of prescription medicine. 'Brain injured' seemed to make sense, it seemed to describe how I felt at the time.

SUNDAY, OCTOBER 1ST, HOLY WATER

Veronica was in a good mood. She wanted to pick my clothes for the day. She picked socks that said, *Good luck socks.* I felt that was fitting. I needed those today!

I wanted to get my truck back from Rocky River Grill, but the paranoid part of me was aware that the truck had been there since Saturday morning. If there really was any kind of conspiracy against me, I was coming up to the 7-day deadline of my life-extension agreement. Leaving my vehicle (still with signage on it) in such a visible and accessible place could make it really easy for them to get to me. There could be a car bomb or the brake lines could be cut . . .

I got my wife (with the kids) to drive me up to Rocky River. I made them drive to the other end of the parking lot. It felt, again, like a suicide mission. I didn't want there to be a car bomb. But I had to do this. I had to find out if I was free and unimportant, or if some of these paranoid feelings had truth to them. This was a test of what was real and what was not.

When I got closer to my truck, I noticed a bit of peanut butter was smeared on the driver's side door.

In the parking space beside me, a car pulled up. There were three guys in the car and one of them was dressed in a suit and looking pretty fancy for 10 a.m. I was just standing there, and they looked a bit uncomfortable with me. I chatted briefly. I vaguely knew these guys. The guy in the suit told me he had been at a wedding the night before. Another car arrived, and there was a quick exchange. Both cars left. It was definitely a drug deal. They were still going strong from the night before.

I wasn't living the same life as them, but I felt closer to them and more accepting of their journey and their struggles than I probably would have been two weeks earlier. As other people were rushing to church, they were chasing something—maybe, in some ways, something similar.

Now, with no one near me, was the time to test. I put the key into the ignition and turned the key. There was no explosion. The music started playing on the radio. The brakes worked.

On the way back from Rocky River Grill, I went to pick up a box of chemicals for my hot tub. The water had a bit of a green colour to it since it hadn't been changed in a while and I had run out of some of the chemicals. It also needed a new filter. The chemicals and new filters had showed online as having been shipped, but they never made it to me. The evening when I landed in Calgary and was starting to really melt down, when it felt like the pressure of work, the world, and my life was crashing down around me, the ex-husband of the candidate I defeated in the nomination race phoned me to say he had my box of hot tub chemicals, that he had found them up at Panorama, the local ski hill resort. At the time, I could not navigate or deal with this. For my last week, the logistics of getting the chemicals, of having to drive up to Panorama, was more than I could handle. Eventually we set up a place I could pick up the lost box in Invermere.

In my old life, soaking in the hot tub for a few minutes was a chance to relax, to let go of some stress, to enjoy some fresh air—a coping mechanism. If I was too busy to get in a morning or evening quick soak, I would be grumpy. It was part of a routine and an attempt to find mindfulness to decompress. It felt like I was leaving behind some problems and some stress in the tub. Having it full of dirty water and not being usable seemed symbolic of the condition of my mind.

It felt amazing to sip on a beer in the sun, pump out the dirty water, and replace it with fresh, clean water. It felt amazing to not be blown up. It felt amazing to not be in the Invermere hospital dying. It felt like I might just have passed the 7-day test. I might just have 41 more years to live! It felt like this clean, fresh water in my hot tub was almost holy.

CHAPTER 9
Medication and Recovery

MONDAY, OCTOBER 2ND

I was taking an increased dosage of medication, and that morning I tried to get back into my regular Monday, Wednesday, and Friday routine of Peloton workouts. The morning workout was incredible, a 30-minute ride led by Ally Love. She seemed like a powerful, sexy symbol of positivity. "Be the boss that you are meant to be," she often says. It filled me with hope that there are good people doing good things.

The playlist with the workout seemed so perfect; the words of encouragement and the messages seemed so symbolic. The bass was pounding, the music pulsed through me. In Vancouver, on the Thursday afternoon, I had gone to Winners and Best Buy to get gifts for the kids, and on an impulse I had purchased some fairly cheap and basic wireless headphones for myself, but the sound quality was really good. These headphones were amazing. There seemed to be little resistance to the pedal strokes. I felt so powerful, I felt like I could pedal so fast, it didn't feel like a workout at all. It felt like a party, like I had taken ecstasy at a rave.

But I knew something wasn't right, the workout was too easy, it was too fun. I realized I had taken some of the quick-release medication a bit before starting the work out.

TUESDAY, OCTOBER 3RD, ANNA

Anna started working for me at the gelati shop when she was in high school. After high school, she came and went from Invermere and working at the gelati shop a number of times. In the fall of 2010, the business was pretty quiet and she was one of my only staff members. The dynamics had shifted from her being an annoying teen brat to us both being young adults in our 20s trying to figure out the world. We had become more like friends and coworkers instead of boss and employee. (Later, Anna helped to set me and my wife up. She was one of the few mutual people both my future wife and I knew at the time.)

Anna and her mom were going to spend all of November, 2010, in Mexico. A lot of Invermere people used to frequent a little town near Puerto Vallarta called Sayulita. I decided to close the shop down for a week and booked a cheap all-inclusive trip to Puerto Vallarta. After a few days at my resort, I made the trip to Sayulita to visit Anna.

Deep down, I thought maybe we would hook up, which of course would have been a mistake. As it turns out, Anna had at least 2 guys into her. It became clear we were definitely not going to hook up. As the night of drinking mezcal continued, I got angry and jealous. There was a small, older bald man dancing by himself, he was drunk or high, but he was happy. And his happiness annoyed me. I pushed him. I wanted to pick a fight. Anna, her friends, and people she knew (including some locals) were quick to defuse the situation, and I never really thought about it again.

The Safe Word is PINEAPPLE!

I had not talked much with Anna in recent memory, but she sent me a Facebook message looking for help on trying to find a place to rent. She opened up about a tough relationship and volatile living situation that she was in. I tried to help, however I could, with finding a rental.

I was in a place of full transparency and oversharing and felt the need to admit that almost 13 years ago back in Mexico I had a crush on her. And then the memory of being an asshole and pushing the old guy came up.

What Anna told me next shocked me: Not only did she already know I was kind of into her back then (more unnecessary guilt and shame I was carrying), but that the old bald guy I had pushed was a gang member. I had been super close to getting stabbed. Anna and her friends literally prevented a stabbing, and I had no idea. It's an interesting perspective on a story that I only knew one side of. And it made me contemplate how many times in our lives are we close to dying or having catastrophic events happen, but we are totally oblivious to it? Even when we know that we were close to being in a traffic accident, or have some vague idea that things could have gone a lot worse, do we really recognize and appreciate just how differently things could have happened? How many times have there been little miracles or flukes that have kept us safe?

The other interesting learning from the conversations with Anna are the gaps in housing supports for women in unstable relationships. The only emergency shelter housing available in Invermere and the area for domestic abuse situations requires a person to literally hide in the safe house and not go to work, give up their pet, and completely disrupt their life. There is no middle ground, no temporary housing options when things have not escalated to a life safety level of severity. And there are no real mental health or counselling supports or services for men, to potentially help to deal with anger and challenges before they escalate into a domestic abuse situation.

I remember a fellow who attended AA explaining to me that you didn't have to hit complete rock bottom to stop drinking and start improving your life. The analogy he used was "You don't have to ride the garbage truck all the way to the dump." I have very little knowledge on emergency housing, but it sure seems like there should be a push to build resources and capacity so that being in a life-and-death situation and having to completely disrupt your life isn't the only way you can access support.

MEDICATION

I was waking up in the middle of the night with cold sweats, my short-term memory was suffering, time was very fluid—too fluid. I was struggling to keep track of which medication I had taken. I think sometimes I was doubling up and sometimes might have skipped a pill, all by accident. I wanted to cut back. The increased dosage felt like too much, like it made things worse, not better.

I told my wife the increased dosage of medication didn't feel right. This did not go well. She was adamant that I should follow doctor's orders. To her, the doctor was God and if he said I needed this much medication, I needed this much medication. We argued about it. I wanted to be honest with her, but I had to also be honest with myself and with what my body was feeling. I decided to start skipping some pills and to keep track of the skipped pills in a separate bag.

We had an unofficial doctor appointment at the Invermere hospital later that day, and my wife and mom attended. I had talked to a friend of a friend who ended up in the Cranbrook psych ward two years earlier, and he strongly recommended taking St. John's wort. It turns out that my family doctor was about to go

The Safe Word is PINEAPPLE!

on vacation to St. John's, and he squeezed in this quick visit at the hospital. My doctor did not seem to be big fan of St. John's wort, and I thought his vacation destination seemed kind of suspicious or coincidental. He confirmed that the cold sweats I was having were a side effect of the medication. He said that there could be some flexibility in the dosage, and then he prescribed more medication, another pill to assist with sleeping, but he said a metallic taste could be a side effect.

I thought that this side effect could potentially be permanent, and it filled me with fear. Enjoying food and hoppy beer brought me so much joy. It reminded me of some kind of Orwellian torture technique, removing all happiness from someone's life. I could not accept a permanent metallic taste.

We talked a bit about how all of this started and the creepy club in Vancouver. My doctor suggested that some of my symptoms and some of my psychosis could have been triggered by drugs, perhaps something in the amphetamine family. Nothing had showed up on the urine and blood tests that they had done, and he suggested that later I might want to get a hair follicle test. Getting drugged at the club would make sense. Bob, the host, had definitely gotten drugged, and the Burger King was a lot of fun and it seemed so profound. I really hadn't slept that night and I felt pretty good the next day, until I didn't . . .

I wanted to get the hair follicle test. I wanted an explanation, but I had to be careful. If I was drugged on purpose and if *they* knew I was getting tested, they might get scared and react, or they could potentially tamper with the test. And there was definitely a chance that all of my online activity and technology usage at home was being monitored. I really had nothing to hide so that didn't matter—except for getting this test. It would be nice to not tip any bad actors onto that.

So I decided to go to the Invermere Public Library and use a computer there to search for hair follicle tests. I bumped into some people I knew, including an agent from my former office. He was kind and supportive, and expressed some concern with how things had been handled.

I filled out an online form for a drug-testing company in Calgary. After returning home from the library, I got a phone call from the company. She told me that I needed to grow my hair out longer, that it had to grow out for around 30 days. The conversation, however, made me uncomfortable. Something about the situation was weird. I wasn't sure if this company was real. It felt like a trap. I googled the lady's name and found an obituary—the person with her name had died a year earlier. This was fucked up!

Around dinnertime, a wave of paranoia hit me really hard. I was really doubting the medication and my doctor. Could I trust my doctor? Could I trust the pharmacy where I got the medication? What exactly was I being prescribed? Technology was so glitchy, I felt like I couldn't trust it. I felt unsafe, even in my own home.

I didn't want to create a scene or draw attention on social media. I didn't want to go to the hospital. I was so sick of feeling this way, I didn't want to be scared, I didn't want to question people anymore. My wife was dealing with putting the kids to bed. I asked my mom, my sister, and the energy-healing neighbour to come over that evening. I trusted all three of them, but just in case there was one of them that couldn't be trusted, the other two would be able to tell.

All three of them have different beliefs and perspectives. I explained my theories and my paranoia. I explained that I felt like I got a second chance at living, some minor version of a "second coming" or something, but that there was the real potential of being persecuted, that it felt like there were these energy waves attacking me and *they*, or some conspiracy, were trying to get to me.

My sister was blunt and unrelenting: I was not the second coming and what I was talking about was crazy. She challenged who "they" were. She pointed out that the names of the lady from the drug-testing company and the obituary were not a perfect match; it was a slightly different name. At my request my mom tried to install a more secure web browser on my computer and researched some of the medication I was on. The energy healer neighbour listened and was kind and calm.

Having the different perspectives and having them at my house helped to calm me down. Overtime, I settled down and the paranoia and anxiety slowly decreased. This was one of the last real waves of paranoia/intense anxiety.

WEDNESDAY, OCTOBER 4TH

The Peloton workout felt hard, like real work. The music was good, but not amazing. Despite the workout feeling harder, my body feeling slower, despite feeling tired and less powerful, my actual output was almost identical to Monday.

During the darkest times, I had this fantasy, this picture in my head, of bobbing on the lake in my new pontoon boat, sipping a beer, bullshitting with a friend or relaxing with the family, with the sun shining. This vision, although at times it seemed impossible to achieve, was motivating. It was one of many tests that I made for myself.

On this day, the weather was perfect, more beautiful and warmer than you would expect for early October. I was feeling stronger. My wife agreed to let me take the boat out, and my friend Justin was available.

I felt so fucking grateful to be alive and to be on that boat with Justin. It felt perfect. I had taken a quick-release pill and drank some beer, so this was definitely contributing to my positive mood. And there was part of me that still thought or felt that I had some special powers. I really believed that I had almost died, and then had 7 days of tests, and now it felt like I had passed. I was getting my old life back, but with enhanced powers, and I might just get 41 more years on Earth to do some good.

Justin was asking about when I was going to winterize the boat, and he was worried about me damaging a prop. I said it didn't matter, I could get a new prop or even buy a new engine. Money felt so unimportant. I felt so rich, not necessarily with money, but with life.

After we got the boat out of the water, I dropped Justin off at his vehicle parked by the Station Pub, where my sister and a friend were on the patio. There was a trivia night, and they invited me to attend. I wanted to, it would have been so much fun. I was cured now, I was good, I was free, I was amazing, and spending the night partying would have been a great way to celebrate not being crazy anymore.

But that would not have made my wife or kids very happy, and I was trying to be a better person, a better father. Either way, I needed to get the boat unloaded. Maybe after the kids were sleeping, if I still felt good, I could ride my bike down to the pub later.

As I pulled away, I yelled out of the window of my truck: "I'm not CRAZY!!! I am just WEIRD!!!"

I really believed it. I thought I was cured.

After some struggles unloading the boat, which again reminded me that this was real life and not some kind of dream, the quick-release medication was wearing off and there was definitely no way I was going out again. I needed to take things slowly. I might be stronger and be getting better, but I definitely wasn't cured yet. I was so glad I didn't stop at the pub on the way home.

THURSDAY, OCTOBER 5TH

Although I was trying to decrease the medication, I knew that I didn't know what I was doing. I tried to see an on-call or fill-in doctor about my prescriptions and dosages, but it sounded like they were booking really far out, weeks out. I saw people in the waiting room at the clinic who looked like they needed the medical care a lot more than I did.

I was going through the quick-release pills pretty fast. I had a prescription for a refill, but I was feeling a bit paranoid about Pharmasave. The last time I went there, a guy who doesn't like me named Glen was leaving the office with Keith the owner. The way that Glen looked back at me, it filled me with chills. If there was any kind of conspiracy against me, this Glen guy would definitely be part of it!

So I went to the other pharmacy in town, one that hasn't changed much since I was a kid. The pharmacist working was patient and calm. I explained that I felt I was over-prescribed with medication and struggling to balance what was the right amount, and at this point I was basically self-medicating and taking less medication.

The pharmacist sat down with me and looked over all of the medication I had been prescribed. She explained to me the difference between slow release and quick release, and I realized that I was definitely taking the quick-release medication when I shouldn't, that taking one slow release in the morning was going to be a much more stable way to medicate versus taking several quick-release pills throughout the day. I asked about the metallic-taste side effect for the sleeping pill, and she explained that could happen briefly while taking the actual pill, but it wasn't permanent.

This little bit of pharmaceutical education, when I was finally in a state to be able to understand it, helped me so much. Switching to the slow-release dosage made a huge difference in avoiding big spikes and crashes from the medication.

Around that time, different people kept asking me: "Are your affairs in order?" This bothered me. What did they know that I didn't? Why was everyone asking me that? Was this some kind of warning? Should I be concerned about my affairs? Should I be concerned about my lawyer? Was he trying to somehow scam some properties or something from me? I was on high alert for any kind of potential persecution and worried about being ripped off.

I went to a different law firm with a crudely typed document I had prepared. I was trying to effectively create some kind of living will. The lawyer and his assistant, both people I had grown up with and trusted, advised against getting this one-page document I had created witnessed. They gave solid advice to check with the law firm I was already using and find out what was on file, to act calmly and not raise any concerns, to not act too crazy.

The lawyer gave great advice with respect to struggling with mental health, indicating that the more irrational someone acts—doing things like trying to take a lot of money out of the bank, trying to make quick legal changes—the more likely a person could lose control of their affairs. And it made sense. A week earlier, I wanted to take out a bunch of cash and potentially be ready to make a quick trip to the West Kootenays or the United States in case I needed to flee from *them*. Luckily, although the threat felt real at times, it never felt that physically present, and being with my kids and following a routine, dealing with locals face-to-face, always made more sense than running away.

I went to my law firm and got them to check the status of my will and power of attorney and so on. It turned out that I had failed to get my mom and sister to sign some legal documents that had been prepared a year earlier. This also made sense, because I think deep down I knew something was unresolved, and when people were questioning me on my affairs, it triggered this feeling.

My mom and sister agreed to sign the documents the next day, and my legal paranoia disappeared.

That day, a story in the local newspaper, the *Columbia Valley Pioneer*, came out, outlining that I was struggling with mental health. Steve, the reporter, was very gracious. I'd ranted to him for 35 minutes on September 29th, when I was still struggling, very vulnerable, scared, and angry. And Steve produced a very kind and gentle story despite my passionate, manic ramblings.

Up until this point, it was only people paying attention on Facebook, or who may have heard through rumours or gossip, who knew that something was off with me. When I was interacting with people around downtown, it seemed like about half the people had followed or heard about my Facebook posts, and the other half had no idea. It was interesting navigating life in a small town, not knowing who knew what.

FRIDAY, OCTOBER 6TH

It was a sunny and beautiful morning. I was having coffee and a bit of food at Stolen Church Coffee, the coffee shop I had founded (originally Gerry's Gelati). The espresso was smooth. It covered my tongue like thick, slightly bitter caramel. Sitting near me was a group of older local guys who meet there most mornings. One of them is a retired realtor. I finished the last bite of my breakfast wrap and asked if I could join their conversation. I told them a tiny bit of my experience, thinking that I was going to die, about the fire alarm, hopefully having 41 more years. I mentioned that I thought I would slowly ease back into real estate.

It was one of the first times I had thought about real estate and my career. Up until this point, it was about surviving, about navigating the paranoia and trying to find out what was really happening, trying to protect my family. But I was starting to feel closer to normal again. I was starting to believe in a bright future again.

Although I wasn't happy with the way that my brokerage had blocked my email and terminated me, I was feeling positive. Maybe I could forgive. Maybe I could work with them to make a new model with real estate, something that had a better work-life balance and where I could contribute back to Invermere and to society. Maybe we could repair the relationship and move forward.

As I was walking down the main street of Invermere, feeling positive, I checked my email on my Samsung phone and found one from the owner of my former office:

> *Good morning, Gerry,*
>
> *We have been asking you to remove your brokerage advertising that includes covering up the brokerage information on your van and removing the decaling from your vehicle.*
>
> *I am now getting complaints about this.*
>
> *I need this addressed right away, Gerry.*
>
> *Thanks for your attention to this matter.*
>
> *Regards,*

I saw red. Part of it was very simple: There was no opening asking how I was doing, and it wasn't framed as a question on how it was going with removing signage. From my perspective, there was no compassion in the message.

I had been in regular communication with the owner of the office and the managing broker. I had already removed brokerage branding online, and I was now finally in a position where I could start to navigate and organize trying to get decals scraped from vehicles and signs covered. But if I was going to go back into real estate, like I had just been thinking about minutes earlier, if there was an opportunity to forgive and make up with the office, what was the point of scraping everything off and ripping things down just to put them back up again? And realistically, everyone in town knew that I wasn't active in real estate at the moment. Whatever bit of branding was out there wasn't directing any real estate business to me; all the emails were going to the office since they had blocked me from my own email.

The feelings of being removed from the office group chat, being blocked from my email, not feeling welcome in the office, the feelings of being instantly cancelled—the emotions came rushing back.

It was so frustrating to think that other agents would be complaining about this stupid signage rule, a rule that the public would have no idea about. And for my office or former office to be so fearful, to cower to the agents threatening to complain. This message, the actions to date, the tone—it pushed me in that moment to decide that I couldn't fully forgive, I couldn't go back. It would be against my new code. It wouldn't be healthy for me.

I went home and wrote an email to the owner of my office and managing broker, expressing my disappointment with the email sent earlier that morning and explaining that I wasn't coming back to the office. I set it to auto send at 3:29 p.m. that afternoon.

I met with the District of Invermere mayor and chief administrative officer that afternoon as well, to talk about going on a medical leave from council. Although I felt like I was doing better, I didn't want to jeopardize any council decisions, and the idea of having a break and not having to sit through some meetings seemed like a good idea.

Although it seemed less likely, there was still part of me that was nervous about what could happen at or near the end of October. I had to spend what time there was enjoying life, being with my family, and trying to write a book, not sitting through boring meetings.

I showed up to the real estate office around 3 p.m. I suspected that the owner and managing broker wouldn't be there, and they weren't. I had about half an hour to clear out my office before the email would hit various inboxes. I quickly emptied the files and items in my desk, and filled several boxes. I removed the art and sales achievement awards from the walls. It hurt to pull down the awards. They had meant so much to me . . .

> *For Royal LePage individual agents not part of team for all Canada for 2022:*
>
> *#10 in all of Canada for units sold*
>
> *#1 in all of BC for units sold*
>
> *#9 in all of BC for commission income.*

I was on track to achieve similar numbers in 2023, and now it didn't matter, I didn't matter—at least not to them. I was now a liability instead of an asset. And I had better get my fucking name scraped off my truck and I had better hurry up and cancel myself. I was mad at them, at the situation, and at myself. I didn't want to be cancelled, I didn't want to be a crazy person. Beneath the anger, there was passion and there was pain. I felt empowered marching out of the office with most of my shit crudely packed up.

On the desk, I had left a bottle of tequila, some business cards, a branded cutting board, my branded jacket, the sales achievement award, and a dead fly I found in a drawer. The combination felt symbolic.

SUNDAY, OCTOBER 8TH

My phone was off or on silent, and I was only checking it every few hours, compared to before when I would literally be glued

The Safe Word is PINEAPPLE!

to it, checking it constantly. When I checked my phone that morning, between 9:01 a.m. to 9:44 a.m., there were four missed calls from a private number and a strange voicemail. The voicemail said something like this: "This the Church of Latter-day Saints and we are doing a survey about crazy people." The voice sounded kind of mean, and the words sounded a bit slurred. Had this call came the week earlier, it would have really triggered me, it could have really started a wave of paranoia. But I recognized it for what it probably was: a weird call, a prank call. I just ignored it.

It was another beautiful day, and I wanted to take the boat back out onto the water. My wife and kids did not want to go on the boat, but they agreed to help me launch it. For the first bit, I floated around by myself. I was one of the only boats on the entire lake and the water was very calm and peaceful. My mind felt calm. I had made arrangements to pick up a fellow named Gurmeet around 3 p.m.

Gurmeet is a polarizing local character. He owns a lot of land in the area. In the 1990s, Gurmeet tried running for mayor and then later tried running for town council; he was unsuccessful on both attempts. He also sued both the town and the school board over different topics. He has been a big critic of past Invermere council decisions, decisions that I was involved in making.

I was trying to build bridges and consider different perspectives. Gurmeet and I haven't agreed on a number of issues, but this felt like an opportunity to rebuild a relationship. The first bit together was pleasant. Gurmeet told some stories about his father in India and about his wife's family. But eventually the conversation got onto topics of past council decisions, specifically around rezoning and development.

It was hard not to take offence to some of his opinions and comments. The conversation started to get heated. Eventually, it turned into a full argument. My theory of considering alternative viewpoints and not being polarized—well, it wasn't perfect, we clearly had different perspectives.

Around this time, Gurmeet paused to pee off the side of the boat. I had the very real urge to push him into the lake, the water was very shallow, but I decided more wisely that it was time to go back to shore. There was a Thanksgiving family dinner at my dad's house, and it was getting close to dinnertime.

When we got close to shore, I realized I needed Gurmeet's help to get the boat out of the water and onto the boat trailer. We had to pivot quickly from arguing to working together. There was a lone man standing in the water fishing, in the middle of the area ideal for loading and unloading boats. He took up a lot of space. I jumped off the boat in the shallow water nearby and backed my truck with boat trailer into the water a safe distance from the fisherman, but the angle wasn't right, the trailer was sideways, and the water wasn't deep enough. I tried going on the other side of the fisherman, but it still wasn't right. He saw me struggling and continued casting his line.

Finally, I very politely asked the man if he would be willing to move out of the way for a few minutes. He looked really annoyed and didn't say anything, but he finally moved over a little bit. I thanked him several times, but he never responded.

The lone fisherman in the water seemed to be another symbol. In one sense, it showed the power of the individual. One person really can have an impact, sometimes just by having strong convictions and by stretching their reach as far as they can. But the power of the individual, if it is not balanced with self-awareness and concern for others, can result in someone who is very rigid, selfish, and objectively an asshole, who can take up more space than they deserve and have negative impacts on others. Perhaps there were times in my life when I had been like the man fishing.

The Safe Word is PINEAPPLE!

TUESDAY, OCTOBER 10TH

I had made the appointment the week before and this was the day the sign shop was available to properly scrape the Royal LePage logo and brokerage name from my truck windows. Although it annoyed me, now that I knew I was done with my former office, it was definitely time to get the signage removed.

One of my goals was to "play more in the dirt" and try to be more hands-on with the rural development I was doing. I had made arrangements to buy a tiny Chinese-made excavator. The guy was driving out from Elkford with the machine, and he wanted me to meet him Cranbrook.

My plan was to grab the dump trailer at the downtown commercial reno project, empty it of construction waste at the landfill, and drive to Cranbrook to pick up the machine. It was an ambitious plan, pushing me beyond my comfort zone and skill level. Trying to strap a tarp over the construction waste wasn't going smoothly, as it took me forever to put various bungee cords and straps across the pile of debris. I was pushing myself to be active and to be normal, to get things done on a deadline, but I wasn't operating at 100%.

Justin showed up with one of his business partners. I didn't really want to see them, because I felt stressed about the timeline and nervous about trying to drive to Cranbrook and transport this machine. And Justin was teasing me. I wasn't in the mood for it.

I got a text message. The guy transporting the mini excavator had left Elkford early; he was going to come the whole way and deliver the machine to my subdivision in Spur Valley. What a relief!

I still had some real estate signage on the side of the road to deal with. I didn't want to rip down the sign and have someone else take the space, and I didn't want to hide my face. I bought a roll of blue duct tape and some garbage bags. I covered up the brokerage name, the words "Buying or Selling?" but I kept my face, website, and cell number visible, and put a big blue "X" through the Royal LePage logo. Technically, that met the rules; there was no more reference to real estate. If people went to my website, it was now only for booking my free community van. I thought the blue duct tape "X" through the Royal LePage logo was funny, but I knew this was edgy. I wouldn't dare post this online.

That evening, I got a very terse email from the owner of the office threatening to take legal action against me for the duct tape cross over the Royal Lepage logo. He was mad. He was hurt. Although I didn't intend it as a personal attack on the owner or the managing broker, they took it very personally.

Initially, I sent the message and some of the correspondence to my lawyer. If they wanted to lawyer up, I would fight them. I was ready for a fight! But I stopped. Did I really want a fight? What was I doing? I had to be honest with myself, was I leading with love and compassion? Was this consistent with my new code? I returned that evening with more black garbage bags and more duct tape. It was raining and windy. Although part of me didn't want to, I covered up the entire sign, even my big ugly face.

It was time to accept responsibility for my situation and to move forward. It was time to live by my code. I was directing the anger, disappointment, and frustration of my entire situation to the office and to the brand, which, realistically, wasn't fair. Could they have shown a bit more compassion and dealt with things better? I think so. But ultimately, was my situation really their fault? I had chosen to take on more work than I could effectively handle, and I (and they) had made a lot of money over the last few years. I had chosen to push to the point of a meltdown, to chase money, to ignore red flags.

And when I didn't know what was happening to me, I had insisted on being public about my experiences, thoughts, and feelings. Oversharing publicly seemed like the best way to protect myself and my family from some kind of conspiracy. But ultimately, it was my choice to be vocal and public. And I had to accept responsibility for my choices and admit when I had gone too far.

My former managing broker said I was "attention-seeking" and acting very selfishly. And when it came to the X over the Royal LePage logo, I think he was right. It was immature, it was dumb. The next morning, I phoned the owner of the office and apologized. I started crying. I was sincere about the apology, and I think he knew that.

Upon reflection, I think that subconsciously I tried blowing up or stress testing everything in my life: my career, my marriage, whether it was even worth being alive. And many things survived, grew stronger, grew in importance. I gained valuable insight and perspective. Unfortunately, there were some casualties; some relationships and arrangements did not survive or were severely weakened. There are regrets and there are pains, there are people I used to be close with who I don't see anymore and who I miss.

CHAPTER 10
Back to the Future

MID-OCTOBER

I slowly decreased the amount of medication I was taking, and by the middle of October I was down to none. I monitored the situation. I felt good, my concentration was much better, my memory no longer fuzzy, and there were no more "energy attacks" or waves of paranoia. I was feeling pretty normal.

During the scary paranoid times, the West Kootenays felt like a safe place; I felt a pull to go there. But I really don't know the area that well. Parts of the West Kootenays I had never visited, like Kaslo. Going to Kaslo and exploring areas closer to home felt both exciting and possible. It wasn't that hard to navigate, and it would be a good test trip with the family to see how we handled travelling.

I was also trying to figure out whether I wanted to rejoin real estate and how to do that. The idea of joining another franchised office, being part of a bigger company and potentially being cancelled or censored again, didn't feel right.

Several years earlier, while we were both briefly serving as directors on the Kootenay Real Estate Board, I met a lady named Jodie, who owns a boutique independent brokerage in Rossland. Jodie started her real estate career at Panorama and had sold some real estate in and around Invermere before moving to Rossland. I reached out to Jodie about the potential to join her office. I wanted to learn the process and procedures of a small independent brokerage, and her business model intrigued me. Jodie was willing to talk, but she was hesitant. She was worried how much of a "loose cannon" I might be. She wanted to meet face-to-face, and she wanted to meet my family and assess how sane and stable I was.

My wife and I decided to plan a weekend trip to the West Kootenays, spend one night in Kaslo, and then the second night in Rossland.

OCTOBER 20TH

My free community van, the GerryVan, was stuck in Saskatchewan. A client had moved there, but it wasn't clear when she was bringing the van back, and it sounded like there were some mechanical problems with the van. Other people were asking to use it. Even though I wasn't licensed for real estate, it felt important to keep the service going. The week before, I had bought a second cube van from a fellow who lived near Moyie Lake. He had delivered the van to Invermere, but there was a glitch with the paperwork. On the way to Kaslo I stopped to get some insurance papers from him. He was an interesting guy, lots of life history and business experience. We chatted for a while.

In Creston, I stopped to look at a big, old, ugly backhoe that was for sale. I wanted to have more time to play in the dirt, I wanted to be more self-reliant with my rural subdivision, and I was definitely feeling a pull towards analog, old-school equipment.

If something crazy were to happen in the Invermere area, having some basic construction equipment could be useful.

OCTOBER 21ST

The feeling of downtown Kaslo, especially the main street retro grocery store, reminded me of Invermere and my childhood in the 1980s. But my wife was grumpy. She complained about the two stops I had made the day before. She thought it took away from family time and that the backhoe was a waste of money. The kids picked up on her mood. Kelvin was being really grumpy, and Veronica was being very difficult. Both kids said that the trip was stupid, and they wanted to be at home.

I got mad. I was trying to spend time with them, I was spending money on hotels and this trip so that they could have a good experience, and I thought it was efficient to do make those two stops along the way instead of making a separate trip. It was normal family tension. Not easy, not always perfect, but not crazy. After we all expressed our frustrations, everyone seemed to calm down. We ended up having a good breakfast. We toured a cool mining museum in the basement of a coffee shop, and Kelvin was very impressed with the huge, old iconic steam wheeler found in Kaslo.

That afternoon, I met with Jodie one-on-one, and that evening, we had a nice dinner with my family and her family.

OCTOBER 22ND

I was sleeping so much better compared to the first week or two after the creepy club in Vancouver, but sometimes I would wake up early. This Sunday morning was one of those mornings. I was browsing what real estate prices and listings were like in Rossland

and Kaslo, when I saw my phone light up. The ringer was on silent, but I could see on the screen "private number."

The creepy calls had continued. The week before, the message that was left on my voicemail went something like: *"Hey, Gerry. We are just doing a quick survey here. I was wondering if you have any bullets? Just a quick 3 questions. First question, are you circumcised? Second question, do you fuck your wife in the ass? And third question is, are you a little pussy ass? Yeah, sorry, sir, this is just a survey to see if you react like a mental patient or not."*

There had been a couple of weird text messages from another number, claiming to be a boyfriend of a local guy, who many think is gay but who refers to his male friends as roommates. Another night there were 12 missed calls between 8:30 p.m. and 10:14 a.m.

I answered the call. An angry voice said, "How dare you send pictures of your dick to my son."

My blood was boiling. "Who is this? I need to know your name."

The man: "Why did you send pictures to my son?"

"I didn't send any pictures to anyone, who are you?"

He said, a bit less angry, "Who are you?"

"My name is Gerry, but I didn't send anything to your son or anyone. What is your name, who am I talking to?"

"Ah, my name is Ken, I'm in Radium. What did you say your name is?"

"Gerry."

"Oh, ah, well I was told your name was Barry."

I said, "I got some weird messages before with someone mentioning Barry. That isn't me."

He said, "Oh, well, ah, that's who it said the photo was from. I am sorry, I mean you know why I would be really angry, right? I mean someone sending that to my son, like that isn't right. Okay, well, thanks for your time."

I didn't know if this was the man who was making all the prank calls, his speech didn't sound slurred, but it was still a weird phone call. But it felt good to answer the phone and stand my ground. I wasn't going to let these calls bother me. There were a few more missed calls, and a few more text messages over the next few weeks. I tried researching the call history with Telus, but they were useless. I mentioned it to an RCMP officer, but he didn't seem interested in looking into it. I let it go.

OCTOBER 25TH

Jodie had agreed to take me on, and I had completed the paperwork to get my real estate licence transferred to her brokerage. The official approval came through on October 25th. I regained access to the real estate database, and I could slowly start rebuilding my career.

Leading up to October 31st, I still had a bit of anxiety about this date. There had been the Hamas attack on Israel on October 7th that led to the Israeli invasion of Gaza on October 27th. Perhaps the vision I had of some ultimate war happening on or before October 31st was some foreshadowing of this conflict. But I didn't think it was. Although I was aware of this terrible situation, it had no direct impact on Invermere and my day-to-day life. Maybe it was a subconscious, self-imposed deadline for getting healthy, a check-in point on my sanity and emotional health.

Initially, I had thought that I could have a book finished and done by the end of October. It was clear to me that was now impossible. But in case there was some significance to the date, I emailed over some draft writing to a mix of contacts and friends before the end of October, just as a bit of a backup, "just in case" move.

OCTOBER 31ST

That evening, the whole family wore matching Waldo sweaters (red and white knitted sweaters my wife had made that look like the character from the *Where's Waldo?* books). We went trick-or-treating in our neighbourhood, and my wife and I alternated handing out candy at home. My wife had heard of a trend: giving out potatoes. We gave out an entire 20 lb. bag of potatoes (along with candy), and the older kids were yelling "POTATO!" and telling all their friends about it. The potatoes were a hit!

The only thing that was odd about the evening was that the managing broker from my former office drove through the neighbourhood, among the crowd of kids and parents. He is older and really had no reason I could think of to be there, and there was no other car traffic. What was he doing? It seemed strange and out of place, but I didn't dwell on it. Weeks earlier, I knew, that could have sent me into a string of paranoid thoughts, but I just let it go. Later, he told me a rental property he manages had an issue with the furnace and he had to drop off a space heater. He was shocked at how busy the neighbourhood was on Halloween and wished he had timed his trip to the rental property differently.

NOVEMBER

The year before, December 2022, we had taken a family vacation outside of San Diego, and we had visited Lego Land California. The sunsets and views of the Pacific Ocean were incredible. It was a fun trip. We had a healthy balance of WestJet dollars, and it seemed crazy to me that I could have almost died with a balance of these unused credits. It was time to have more experiences and to take another family trip!

My wife had always wanted to go to Universal Studios, and the kids were excited about the idea. I wanted sunshine and ocean views. We booked a trip, flying into LA, renting a car, staying in a hotel near Redondo Beach, and spending two days at Universal Studios. We were flying out November 19th. It was something to look forward to.

On November 8th, I sent out an email to local realtors explaining that some of my experience may have been triggered by accidental drug exposure, that I was now licensed with the boutique brokerage in Rossland, and that I was looking forward to re-entering real estate and working collaboratively with everyone.

I still wanted to know whether I had been drugged. So, on November 13th, I visited the drug-testing company in Calgary. The lady who I had previously feared was dead—or part of some kind of trap—was definitely alive. She snipped some hair from the top of my head and slid it into a plastic sample bag and sent it to the lab for a 15-panel hair follicle drug test.

On November 15th, I got a call from my new managing broker. It sounded like the Interior Association of Realtors had received several complaints against me. Tears filled my eyes. I felt so defeated, so tired, so helpless. It had been such a struggle over the last month and half, and although I felt like I had made some real progress from the middle of October to the middle of November, things were still very raw and I was still very vulnerable. This hit me hard. At first, Jodie thought she heard that some of the complaints were coming from agents in my former office. That didn't make sense; I couldn't picture that being true (it wasn't). The uncertainty of what the complaints were about, and who was making them, was almost unbearable. The information slowly trickled out over the course of the next 2 weeks.

The trip to California was fun and pleasant. We successfully navigated driving through LA traffic, and I got to visit some iconic places I had always wanted to see, like Santa Monica and

Long Beach. The kids had fun playing in the ocean, and there were some beautiful sunsets. But I had these underlying feelings of fear, anxiety, anger, and a general helplessness as it related to the complaints. Not knowing all the information, not knowing if this would block me from restarting my real estate career or if this would push my new managing broker to decide I was too much trouble and drop me—it was hard to not worry about these things.

One of the agents who filed a complaint had suggested to the real estate board that I take six or more months off before relicensing. It seemed ridiculous to me that people who had never taken the time to talk to me directly, who had no idea what emotional and mental condition I was currently in, who had no idea about my journey of recovery, and who have no medical training, could come up with "solutions" for me and could have any influence over me attempting to rebuild my career.

Jodie really stepped up and helped to advocate for me. There were several phone calls and emails. Around the middle of December, the complaints were withdrawn.

On November 29th, I received an email: The results were back from my hair follicle drug test. Maybe I am one of the only people who has ever taken a drug test and was hoping for a positive result. It felt like something weird happened at that creepy club, and proving that I had been drugged would have helped to explain so much of what happened to me and so much of my breakdown. Using my phone, I quickly logged into the account to access the details. I skimmed the one page, on the far-right column under the category "Results" for all 15 drug categories. The word "negative" repeated over and over. I was disappointed. Prior to my breakdown and the creepy club, I had been regularly vaping marijuana, so it had seemed strange that even this result was negative.

Later that day, I complained to Justin about the results. As I was talking to him, I reopened the results on my desktop computer. Looking closer, it was interesting to see that for almost all of the drug classes under the "Confirmation Cut Off" column, the results showed "none pg/mg" but for amphetamine and cannabis (THC), the amount was blank (but the end result still showed negative). I believe for those two classes of drugs, there were some traces found, but the amounts were below the screening cut-off level (I believe the cut-off level is set to avoid false positives, to account for environmental factors).

I did some googling (I won't call it research). It sounds like hair follicle tests are more reliable at detecting regular, long-term usage of drugs but less reliable for occasional use or one-time exposure to certain drugs. I could have been exposed to something in the amphetamine family, but, ultimately, the drug results were inconclusive.

CHAPTER 11
Learnings, Conclusions, and Reflections

SUMMER 2024

There have been minor ups and downs, some beautiful moments, stressful moments, but generally a lot of normal. My family is doing well, not perfect, but we never were. I have been seeing a counsellor and an energy healer. I have been writing and recounting the events. The fear, the anger, the pain of my experiences have shifted into learnings and realizations. I have come most of the way to a place of acceptance for the outcomes—both positive and negative—of my breakdown (although there are regrets, and parts of it are painful to revisit).

I think my experience will make me a better person, a stronger, more compassionate person, and I think it will help me to dedicate my time and energy to the right directions for the next 41 years (or hopefully more). But I wouldn't go so far as to say I'm glad it happened, or glad it happened the way it did. Ideally, these learnings could have come in a less dramatic way, a way that was less stressful and scary for my family, friends, and community. Ideally, others can come to these learnings in a healthier way.

It was a slow initial restart to my real estate career, over the late fall of 2023 and early winter of 2024. Initially, I wasn't ready for too much. It is so heartwarming and reassuring that many past clients and locals are reaching out to list their properties and to trust me with real estate sales. I am hoping to put in some new systems, add some admin support, and delegate some work to avoid a repeat of taking on too much work.

I have made a point of revisiting places—Vancouver, the hotel, and the hotel restaurant in Calgary. I haven't gone to the creepy club or the Granville Street Burger King yet. Maybe someday. It has been amazing to see some elected -official friends and UBCM executive and staff members in person at several conferences in 2024. They have all been so loving and accepting.

POLARIZATION AND CONSPIRACIES

When you are running down the street of your neighbourhood with your daughter in your arms, and you are questioning whether you are alive or in a coma, when you are not sure what is real, but all you want is a neighbour to protect your child and for people to witness that you would never hurt anyone, in that moment, you do not give a flying fuck who your neighbours voted for or what their opinions on vaccines are.

It feels like polarization is increasing. We are being pushed into picking sides, being divided into groups, and being pushed into fighting each other. Whether this is purposely being driven by evil forces or whether it is an accidental by-product of the human condition and the algorithms of social media, I don't know, and I don't know if it matters.

In an emergency, in a moment of need or panic, these political identities really don't matter. What does matter is family and community, and the very real human desire to help each other. I think we all have a role to play in pushing back against polarization.

The visions of black eyes and white eyes, good people and bad people, was far too simplistic. Almost everyone will view themselves as being close to, or completely, on the good side; very few people will identify with being evil. Even if we know some of our actions are bad, we almost always have justifications for these actions.

The reality is that I think most of us are grey people, floating between good and bad. Embracing and accepting that we are all flawed and imperfect can help us with not viewing other groups of people as being evil or bad and can avoid us from worshiping or idolizing or envying others who we perceive as being perfect or virtuous.

When we focus on high-level concepts, when we focus on shared values, we end up having so much more in common with each other. We might not agree on the finer details, or we might make different conclusions/connections (or use different language to describe the same things), but it really doesn't matter. Arguing or caring about finer details that are impossible to prove one way or the other is such a silly way to spend scarce time and energy, and such an easy way to damage relationships and connections.

I was convinced some evil people were messing with me. Everything from YouTube videos and text messages to glitchy technology was giving me clues and evidence to support my theories, beliefs, and feelings. When we view society as being controlled by certain evil forces, we will seek out or notice evidence to support our theories. If you think that you control your own destiny and can manifest certain things to happen in your own life, you will also find evidence to support this belief. When bad or unfair things happen to us, or when the rules of society and economic realities are stacked against us, I think most of us are very quick to look for justifications, someone to blame and to search for patterns or answers, to find meaning in the chaos.

Whether it is the law of attraction, confirmation bias, or some kind of karma, deep down we know that what we think, what we feel, what our beliefs are, how we act and react to others, what we put out into this world—that this all has some impact and connection to what we receive back from the world and from other people.

I had judged and criticized conspiracy theorists like my mom, yet when I didn't know what was happening and I felt like I had lost all control, I was quick to adopt or invent my own conspiracy theories to help make sense of things and to shift the blame and responsibility to someone or something else.

TRIGGERS, BEING MISUNDERSTOOD, AND LISTENING

We are so quick to view so many actions or inactions by other people as personal slights against us, or to try to make someone else's situation about us. And, more often than not, those triggers, those things that we interpret as attacks or slights from other people, they are unintentional and often accidental.

And when we have made mistakes, done or said things we regret, we often hold so much guilt and shame for these past mistakes. But realistically, it is very common that other people have forgotten, never noticed, or have forgiven us long ago. Guilt and shame are heavy, they wear us down. They give other people power over us.

Being misunderstood, having people not accept or believe you, or having people not recognize your true motivations—these are some of the most painful triggers for me. The fear of being judged, of not being accepted, it holds us back from being vulnerable, from being honest. Deep down, we are all still little kids who want to be heard, seen, and loved.

If we can understand, accept, and love ourselves, even our flaws, the triggers don't trigger as much. Our identities, our stories about ourselves, our ego, are not as delicate. We are not as easily "attacked." We are better able to recognize how hurt and fucked up the people who are trying to push buttons, who are intentionally attacking, really are.

We need to build the capacity, time, and skill of listening into our personal relationships, but also into our community, society, and government systems. So many services and institutions are very difficult to navigate, and we know that so many people are already on edge and easily triggered. When the first point of contact is a big sign that says "harassment will not be tolerated" and the people seem to only be interested in or only able to fill out checklists, a human element is missing. When systems lead with fear and anger, it shouldn't be a surprise if people react with fear and anger.

In some of my most manic periods, what I really wanted from the health care system was someone with even a basic amount of training who would listen. I wanted and needed genuine human connection, love, and compassion. I got some amazing treatment, and I did get some genuine care, but it was barely enough. If I wasn't as privileged as I am, if I had a history of mental health issues or a criminal record, if I had reacted more angrily, if I had shown any violence, my story and my experience—and my recovery—would be very different.

There are many lonely and isolated people. If they could be listened to, or even be encouraged and empowered to become a listener, I think that our families and communities would benefit. What if hospital emergency rooms had designated listeners available to just hear people, available to give hugs and human connection? What if, instead of putting security guards into uniforms, we put them into regular clothes and gave them counselling training? I think it would save lives and improve health care outcomes.

BUREAUCRACY, POLITICAL CORRECTNESS, AND DOUBLESPEAK

In an effort to improve safety, to create fairness, we have allowed our regulations and systems to become more and more complex. The analogy I love is that of a Christmas tree with a lot of decorations: We keep adding more and more decorations, to the point that not only does the tree not function as a beautiful Christmas tree (since it is now an ugly mess of crap), but it's also about to collapse with the weight of stuff we keep putting on it. We need to rethink some of our rules, regulations, and government systems; we can't just keep adding rules on top of rules.

Bigger and more centralized systems rarely improve efficiencies and human experiences. The more disconnected people are from the decision-making and the less influence they feel in the process, the less trust and buy-in they have.

There is real value to having more transparent and local decision-making. There is real value in having more personal responsibility and not having to rely on a central government or system for basic needs. I believe that Canada has a very transparent political system, and I don't think there is much corruption among elected officials. I do, however, wonder or fear whether there could be corruption (or just incompetence) within the public sector. There are bureaucrats who wield an immense amount of power and control, and there is very little transparency or oversight to make sure that things are being administered in a fair, efficient, and logical way.

We need to push against overly complex systems, onerous regulations, and unnecessary centralization. Complexity can be used as shield to hide inaction or inefficiency. It prevents transparency, it hurts public trust and engagement. Simplicity and common sense encourage transparency, action, and accountability.

I believe we need our leaders and our governments to speak in honest, transparent, and blunt terms. We should not have two sets of language: one that is official, polite, and says almost nothing and means nothing, and a second for how real people actually talk to each other. Part of the reason that Donald Trump and some right-wing politicians are so popular is because they talk like regular people and they say things that regular people think. Candid, real talk shouldn't only belong to the extreme right wing.

IT'S INSIDE YOU

One of the scariest times in my life was in the hotel restaurant in Calgary on Saturday, September 23rd—the gloom, the anxiety, the dread, admitting that I was 1% suicidal. But when I really focused, I had clarity: *You know what you need to do, you just need to do it.* I think for most of us, this is true. We might not listen, we might not like it, often we don't actually do it, but deep down, we usually know what we need to do.

I no longer believe that I have any special powers (or am any kind of demigod or second coming). I now doubt that there was any conspiracy against me. It seems more and more that the visions and realizations I made when negotiating an extension of my life are likely ideas that came from within.

Did I almost die and negotiate to extend my life? Probably not literally, but figuratively and emotionally, I still choose to believe it. I gained valuable insight. I took my mortality seriously, and I learned a lot. Part of me died, and part of me was reborn.

My biggest learning is the power of being honest with myself. When you are honest with yourself and you accept your flaws and past mistakes, it gives you the power to drop shame and guilt.

Dropping shame and guilt allows you to lead with love and compassion, which makes it easier to be vulnerable. And when you are vulnerable, people are vulnerable back. Trust and relationships strengthen.

This will remain my personal code of conduct and will continue to be the contract I have with myself for the rest of my life. Maybe it is something others can consider adopting in their lives:

- Family has to come before community; I need to focus on my kids first.
- I will try not to lie to myself.
- I will try not to lie to others, but I accept that they may not always be ready for my full truth.
- I will ask for consent first. I will not force my views or ideas onto other people.
- I will never intentionally harm myself or anyone else, but I am not responsible for other people's feelings and triggers (offending someone is not necessarily harming them).
- I will lead with love and compassion, not fear and anger.
- I will try to drop all shame and guilt.
- I will have faith in my neighbours and my community, but even if they fail me, my love for Invermere is unconditional.
- I will work on ideas to improve society and systems, but my focus is Invermere. I am not responsible for fixing everything, I cannot control the outcomes, I am not responsible for saving the world.
- I will put limits on how much I work and how much money I make.
- I will never be worshiped; I am a flawed human, not a god.
- I will have more fun!

Even when the answers are usually within us, there are times when, despite doing everything right and giving it our full and complete effort, it can feel like the world is against us. It can be

The Safe Word is PINEAPPLE!

too much to navigate. It can be completely overwhelming, and it can be necessary to let go of control, to give in and give up, to admit that we need help.

I hope that we can build families, communities, and societies where people have full and complete faith that if they need help, if they yell "PINEAPPLE!" (or however they ask for help), there will be real-life angels (family members, neighbours, friends, strangers, health care professionals) who can lead with love and compassion, who can listen, and who can support.

And I hope that those of us who have lived through wild mental and emotional experiences, who are recovering, who have benefited from receiving support, will be able to share our experiences, our stories, and our realizations. The more we share and the more we work on practical solutions, the less being honest and transparent will be met with judgements and negative outcomes.

I see you, I hear you, I love you.

With love and compassion, your flawed (and kind of crazy) friend,

Gerry

ACKNOWLEDGEMENTS

Thank you to anyone who has taken the time to read this story and think about the concepts.

A huge thank you to my immediate family. To my wife, I know you think writing this book was a dumb idea and I know you are pretty much always right… thank you for quietly supporting me on yet another project. To my kids, I love you so much and it was so worth the fight to spend more time with you and to understand you better. To my sister, you had the perfect balance of patience/support and realism. To my mom, you were there, like always, dropping everything and offering complete unconditional love, thank you. To my dad, I know you were scared and worried and that means you care. To Tommy & Joan, thanks for being around and being supportive. All of you are a huge part of my life. You were there for me during the scariest moments; you let me retain freedom. You had faith that I would figure shit out.

Thank you to my friends for the support, for the love, and for the pushback. Many of you were subjected to some terrible writing and weird emails during the process. Some of you are named in the book, I figured you could handle it (and vaguely asked permission, I think). For others, it didn't feel right to specifically name you. Clearly this book is from my perspective, and some creative liberties were taken, not all events or people are exactly as portrayed—something like that (don't sue). Some of you might have different memories and perspectives, and I encourage anyone and everyone to share their own stories.

Thank you to fellow Invermere town council members and senior staff at the District of Invermere, and key executive and staff members with the Union of British Columbia Municipalities—thank you for listening and thank you for not shunning or "cancelling" me, this helped so immensely to my recovery.

Thank you to the general community of Invermere & area. For the people who gave hugs, who sent heartfelt online messages, who opened up about their struggles or struggles in their families. It means a lot. We are stronger together and we shouldn't be afraid to have these kinds of open, honest, and vulnerable conversations.

For editing, concept development, and help with the writing process, there are so many people who played a role but a specific and big thank you to some of the published authors and professionals, who I am happy to call friends, and who helped immensely along the way, including: Dauna Ditson, Margo Talbot, Tony Berryman, and Friesen Press Editor Claire Matthews.

Writing a book really is tough, and you helped make it a bit less hard!

Printed in the USA
CPSIA information can be obtained
at www.ICGtesting.com
LVHW091236260924
791981LV00013B/810

9 781038 316806